TRUE HEALTH, THE INSIDE JOB

Kat Elton

Also By Kat Elton

A Resilient Life: Learning to thrive, not just
survive, with rheumatoid arthritis

TRUE HEALTH, THE INSIDE JOB

Kat Elton

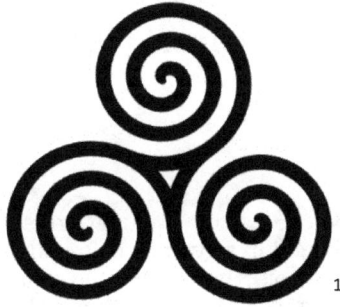

---

[1] "Triple Spiral." Triple Spiral. Symbols.com, n.d. Web. 28 May 2015.

True Health, The Inside Job, by Kat Elton

Copyright @ 2015 by Kat Elton

Printed in the United States of America

Book Cover/Interior design by Jarran Design

ISBN 978-0-9906-8900-3

Library of Congress Number: 2014917129

For all the people who helped me along the way

And for Todd, for understanding

TABLE OF CONTENTS

PROLOGUE

The art of living is a skill to be honed. People will debate endlessly about the right way to live, what is acceptable, the definition of success, and how to behave, but the bottom line is this; a prescriptive life is never a healthy one.

A healthy life can only be found when you begin to have the gumption to dig deep inside, stop listening to others opinions, and begin to walk on your own path. Once this happens you will be led to a different life than the one you are living now.

Ultimately, we all have similar needs and desires: to be loved, to belong, to provide for ourselves and our loved ones, and to have freedom. But every one of us has a life that is unique in its gifts and challenges. Each has value and will help us to grow into the person we are meant to become. Along the way we will change as we grow, and if we are paying attention we will become more skilled. Challenges can bring the skills of courage, resilience, strength, acceptance, gratitude, compassion, and empathy. Over time our challenges will teach us how to meet them well and how to have deep gratitude for the gifts we have been given.

True health cannot be seen; it can only be felt. Honing the skills that life teaches you will lead you to the place inside where true health resides. Only then will you discover the fountain of health; one that defies any setback life hands you, any disease that you find yourself living with, any pain that you have. You will be healthy, life regardless.

INTRODUCTION

What is health? This is a question I began to ask myself five years ago. I was diagnosed with a chronic, incurable disease at age two and I'd always viewed myself as someone who was ill. No matter what I did or how I felt, the label of juvenile rheumatoid arthritis stuck to me like flypaper. For the first thirty-three years of my life I dealt with my fate one of two ways. I either sucked it up and tried to be the "good patient" and uncomplaining daughter, friend, girlfriend, and sister, or when I felt good enough I tried as hard as I could to run away from it, literally, by working my body hard and spending time with people who thought three-hour bike rides up a mountain pass were just another day in the great outdoors. Inside my sunny façade, though, I felt doomed and hopeless about my circumstance. I knew that even if I could fool some people into thinking that the arthritis was no big deal, the truth was that there was a faceless monster inside chasing me down and trying to cripple my body and soul. I believed that despite my best efforts it would always win.

I believed this because that's what I'd been told. Not literally, but clearly enough in the looks of the doctors I saw throughout my life, the whispered comments I'd hear behind my back, and the treatment from others. On days that the pain and swelling got the best of me I'd hear cheery words like, "It'll get better soon, you're doing great," come out of the mouths of people around me, but their body language was clearly stating, "Get me as far away as I possibly can, I don't want to see this." Illness up close can be too stark of a reminder of human frailty, especially when it is in the form of a young child.

So the monster chased me down, sometimes turning up in dreams, always in my psyche, and I responded by isolating myself from others. This wasn't completely apparent, even to myself; I did my best to appear connected, but I protected myself from true connection. As a youngster I did this by telling people what I knew they wanted to hear, and as a young adult by choosing relationships with men who were so self-interested that their curiosity about really knowing me was extremely limited.

This modus operandi lasted until it took too much energy and my body collapsed. I ended up sicker than I'd ever been and unable to hide anything from anyone. Any platitudes that I could come up with fell on deaf ears because my dire situation was too obvious. One day I realized that I couldn't take a bath to ease my pain because I wouldn't be able to get out. I had sequestered myself far away from family who could help and the only significant other I had was an ex-boyfriend who drained me with his need. I suddenly understood that I truly had become what I'd always tried to run from. I'd become ill.

It took me many years to climb out of my abyss and I know that on some level it will always be my life's work, but in the process I finally came to know the truth about health. Health has nothing to do with whether you have been diagnosed with a disease.

Health is found in the answer to these questions:
- Are you living an authentic life?
- Are you able to have unfettered honesty in your relationship to yourself?
- Are you your own best friend?
- What do you really need to be content?

Health is found in the path of least resistance, learning to move towards what you want instead of against what it is that you don't. True health, despite what we've been led to believe, is more about letting go than adding. It requires you to stop re-reading the last chapter of your life so you can start the new one. Eventually the quest for health becomes the search for the truth of who you are. Once your life begins to genuinely reflect this truth, health follows.

Throughout this book, I'll lead you through what I've learned during my quest toward health and guide you on yours. It won't be easy, but is your life easy now? True healing requires great change, immense commitment, unrelenting perseverance, and dogged determination. For healing to happen there has to be a conscious decision and the knowledge that you won't end up getting back to your old self. Instead you will become who you were truly meant to be. The birth of healing begins with the commitment to yourself that you will do the work required. You will never give up, and you will keep hope alive. You are guaranteed through your efforts to move towards health. You are stronger than you know. So together, let's begin walking this road. The first step is to believe that you can.

BELIEF

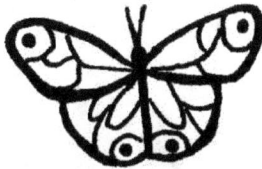

"Live your beliefs and you can turn the world around."

- Henry David Thoreau[2]

[2] Henry David Thoreau quote. (n.d.). Retrieved from
http://www.brainyquote.com/quotes/quotes/h/henrydavid379353.html

The field of quantum physics has changed what we know about the world for those people who are paying attention, and the implications for healing are too important to ignore. What scientists have discovered is that at the subatomic level quantum particles exist as potentials until they are observed. To explain this in another way, in the tiny realm of the smallest amount of a physical entity that can exist, there are little vibrating packs of energy that can't be fully understood. These packs of energy hang out sometimes as particles, sometimes as waves, with no definite location, as if they haven't decided what or where they want to be. They do this until someone, like a scientist taking measurements, causes them to settle into something. The observer actually brings the observed object into being. To make one's head spin even more, at the quantum level there is something called non-locality. This means that tiny quantum particles can influence each other instantaneously even if they are separated by great distances. Hard to fathom but true: the speed of light is not the speed limit of the universe.

These findings are astonishing to think about. Nothing exists independently of our perception of it. Every minute of every day we are creating our reality. Energy is influenced and influences other energy across vast space and without regard to time. It's the butterfly effect happening everywhere all at once. We really are all connected. We are weaving the web of life together all the time.

Medical science has still not caught up with the ramifications of these astounding truths. The idea of evidenced-based medicine would implode if medical researchers admitted to the fact that just by creating an experiment with the expectation of an outcome, the outcome is influenced. The pharmaceutical industry is already grappling with the problem of the placebo effect, or the fact that during clinical trials new drugs often don't perform better than sugar pills. Between 20-60 percent of the time, just expecting that a pill will help will do the job of making you feel better. There is a good argument made by medical historians that the history of medicine is the history of the placebo effect, since for most of history doctors did not have accurate knowledge about how to treat disease. Having a doctor who listens, has the intention of healing, and believes that he or she can help you can be just as effective as one who has access to the latest available treatments in many cases.

Medical science as we know it right now has invested much in the idea that the physical body is similar to a machine and can be tested, measured, sliced and diced, taken apart and put back together. Medicine gets so much messier when you have to take into consideration a person's thoughts, feelings, beliefs, and environmental influences. Frankly, there just isn't enough time for that. When you take an honest look at modern medicine you come to realize that it is just as sick as the people it treats. It is filled with ego, motivated by profit, rigid in its thinking, disdainful of any other healing system, based on a caste system in which the doctor is God, and resistant to change. Medicine right now has little to do with the search for truth and a lot invested in maintaining the status quo.

Perhaps this is because the Western world values reason over emotion, and places a lot of value on logic. Medical science thinks it can out-smart illness, and is on the eternal quest for a magic bullet to cure each disease. Conquering disease is the theme that permeates medicine, to be accomplished through new technology and new drugs. This inflated view of the powers of the scientific method completely ignores the new understanding of how the world works and other ways to influence healing. Medicine has become a Don Quixote, hanging on to its altered perceptions about its power and forcing patients to join it on its adventures.

Not too long ago I woke up from a deep sleep with the thought, "My rheumatoid arthritis is a ghost. What is arthritis anyway?" The word arthritis is made up of components that mean joint (arth) and inflammation (itis). This is describing my symptoms, not telling me what causes them. Okay, how about rheumatoid arthritis is an autoimmune disease? This just means that the immune system is attacking the cells of the organism producing them (that would be me.) Again, this describes what is happening, not why.

"Well then," I thought, "What about the medicine the doctors use to help me? Aspirin must be REALLY good, after all eighty million pounds of it are consumed every day. I took about twelve aspirin a day for the first seventeen years of my life; did the doctors know of some secret ingredient that was healing me?" Actually, no, aspirin works to decrease chemicals in the body which increase inflammation, thereby managing symptoms. When I examined some of the exciting new drugs for rheumatoid arthritis I discovered this; Enbrel decreases the chemical messengers that increase inflammation, as do Humira, Kineret, Remicaide, and more. Methotrexate, the gold standard drug for my disease, interferes with the production and maintenance of DNA. It isn't known how it works, just that it does. This doesn't sound promising to me. I realized that I've been enmeshed in a system of healing for forty years that has no idea how to heal me. All this time they had been giving me internal band-aides to keep my symptoms at bay. My "disease" is really just a name for some symptoms. The real culprit is a ghost, an unknown entity.

It won't take an inquiring mind long to find mountains of information about healing beyond the bounds of Western medicine. Healing cam happen through the Chinese practice of Chi Gung, the Japanese Reiki system, Native American shamanic ceremonies, Peruvian San Pedro rituals, and Christian prayer. These systems of healing have more to do with the quantum model than with the medical model because they are based on the idea that energy can influence matter.

Ultimately, we all choose whom to believe about everything, and these beliefs end up creating our reality. For much of my life I'd been influenced into thinking that my only option was to go to a doctor and take medication, when in fact I had so many more options available to me. Belief is so important because it creates the fabric of our life. An important question to always ask yourself, especially when it comes to your health is, "Whom do I believe?" True health begins when you turn your ingrained beliefs on their head, shake out all the debris, and then put them back in consciously one at a time. Think it of a spring-cleaning for your belief system. Questioning everything that has been given to you as truth and then listening to your inner guidance is one of the most profound things a person can do on their quest for health.

Questioning and shifting my beliefs altered the lens through which I viewed my life, and over time began to transform the shape of my life. As I no longer believed that I was proving my value by working at a five-day-a-week job, I was able to simplify and give my body the rest it needed to feel good. When I "came out of the closet" about my belief in energy medicine, homeopathy, essential oils, Reiki, and other non-conventional healing practices, I felt free to incorporate them into my life without hiding. Once I did this, suddenly I attracted people who were completely accepting and at ease with this lifestyle, not judgmental and patronizing. By relaxing into the ups and downs that my disease brings me instead of trying to figure them out all the time, I stopped wasting my precious energy and began to feel more at ease even when my pain level was high. I was able to leave my house and happily move in with friends once I accepted the fact that a huge amount of the daily stress I felt was caused by the upkeep of a big yard and house that I didn't need. I no longer believed that this house was essential to a good life, to being a successful adult. With each shift, I felt more relaxed. Like a snake shedding its skin as it grows, I cast off long-held assumptions about who I was, and in the process became a healthier version of myself. I finally knew, deep in my core, that my health was my choice, not a byproduct of fate, luck, or DNA. I could choose to be healthy through my belief and through the actions this belief created.

Whenever I need inspiration I think of Anna Mae Bullock, who was born dark skinned in 1939 in Nutbush, Tennesee. As a youngster she was put to work beside her parents as a sharecropper. She was kicked out of the house at age 18 after she became pregnant, and moved in with her grandparents. She married, at age 22, a man who physically and emotionally abused her, and stole her money to maintain his cocaine habit. After years of abuse and a particularly awful fight, she left him with 37 cents in her pocket and hid for months fearing for her life. She paid off debts working multiple jobs. She never gave up. She believed in herself even when those around her were trying their best to knock her down. She is renowned internationally for her singing career, has multiple Grammy Awards, has been inducted into the Rock and Roll Hall of Fame, and has a star on the Hollywood Walk of Fame. She is Tina Turner.

What if young Tina had chosen to believe her parents when they told her she was a disgrace because she became pregnant? What if she believed Ike when he told her she would never get anywhere without him? Where in the world did she find the courage to leave Ike with 37 cents in her pocket? How did she know that she'd be okay? Maybe what she knew was that by believing what she'd been told her reality would never change. She'd always be her husband's punching bag and the focus of her parents' judgment. Maybe their truth didn't feel right to her deep inside. Maybe she knew that she would be able to move into a better future only if she believed enough in herself to take the first step.

"A journey of 1,000 miles begins with a single step." –Lao Tzu[3]

That first step is always the hardest. Believing in yourself and a better future comes with its risks. What if you fail? What if you work very hard, believe in yourself and your ability to heal, and nothing changes? For many years these questions plagued my thoughts and battled with the hope that I tried to create inside. I'd heard of miracle healings happening in places like Lourdes, France, and spontaneous remissions witnessed by uncomprehending doctors, but when I dared to hope that healing was possible for myself I'd quickly feel doubt creep inside. I'd remember the times in the past when I'd dare to hope and had my hopes dashed.

Hope had become a loaded word for me. I HOPE I'll feel good on vacation. I HOPE the pain won't make my bike ride hard. I HOPE I won't limp on the first date I have planned. I HOPE that the medication I have to take will help me more than hurt me. I HOPE that someday I will have a day free from pain.

HOPE: to cherish a desire with anticipation; to desire with expectation of obtainment; to expect with confidence.

Be careful what you hope for, I always told myself, because beyond hope can lie disappointment and heartbreak. How long can you hold onto hope before it dies a slow death?

Hope against hope: to hope without any basis for expecting fulfillment.

So I began to hope against hope. I HOPE someday the arthritis will let go of me. Hah! Good luck. Trying that on for awhile, I sank into a mire that felt horrible.

Like it or not, a life with pain keeps my hope alive, because without it I have nothing. I've finally realized that you never can have too much hope. Hope is life. As the Latin proverb says, "While I breathe, I hope." Despite the outcome, hope always feels good. In the end that was good enough for me and what led

---

[3] L., & Lau, D. C. (1963). Verse 64 Line 10. In Tao *te ching*. Baltimore: Penguin Books.

me to finally take the first step. I took a vow to myself, to believe in myself and my ability to be the person I was meant to become. As Goethe says, trust yourself and you will know how to live. I found myself constantly asking myself, "What am I doing?" and "Why am I doing this?" If the answer involved assuaging an anxiety or acting out of fear I'd stop and switch gears. Over time, I began to make choices that more closely reflected my belief in myself and my ability to heal. If everything really is energy, the way the quantum physicists say, then wasting energy on self-defeating thoughts is not a good idea. If you are trying to become healthy from the inside out it makes much more sense to choose beliefs that empower you. I must admit though, this road is long.

"Hope is the thing with feathers that perches on the soul, and sings the tune without words, and never stops at all."
-Emily Dickenson[4]

It's easy to believe in the things that you are validated for every day. I have some very beautiful friends and if I say, "Wow, you look great today!" it wouldn't be a stretch for them to believe me. If you get A's in school, it's not hard to believe that you are smarter than the average Joe. My friend Tim, who can ride circles around me on his bike, doesn't have to be convinced that he is in good shape. But believing in yourself when life hasn't shown you what you need to see to believe takes courage. How can you hold onto belief when you are trying to create a new reality for yourself? When there is no one to say, "Oh yeah, I can see that in you." What makes a person decide to believe in themselves at all costs?

I think that the reason life sometimes throws us into the gutter is so that we can finally wake up and decide to believe in ourselves enough to change. What if Ike Turner hadn't been mean to Tina? Would she have stayed working as a back-up singer her whole life, never realizing her full potential? At one point the famous country singer Willie Nelson's career was so bad that he found himself lying on the middle of a road waiting to die. What if this hadn't happened? Would he have had the courage to say to himself, "I'm too miserable trying to be someone else, I might as well try being myself." Would he still be there, plucking his guitar to someone else's tune? If my

---

[4] Emily Dickinson quote. (n.d.). Retrieved from
http://www.brainyquote.com/quotes/quotes/e/emilydicki154102.html

disease hadn't decided to hit me with a vengeance at the prime of my life, I know I would still be a strict internal taskmaster and my own worst enemy in many ways. I would still be trying to be successful in the manner that was laid out for me when I was young. Sometimes you have to lose everything you hold precious before you can find the gumption to shoot for the moon.

"All great truths begin as blasphemies." –George Bernard Shaw[5]

So, what do you do after you've said to yourself, "I can do this," but before you've gotten good at actually doing it? When your whole life is based on the faith that you can, even when your external world doesn't yet reflect this? This is when you learn to become a dreamer. To begin believing in infinite possibilities. And to seek out the miraculous. If you spend time looking, there are a lot of unexplained and amazing things to be found. Tibetan Lama Phakyab Rinpoche was ordained by the Dalai Lama when he was thirteen as the Eighth incarnation of the Phakyab Rinpoche. He emigrated to the US in 2003 as a refugee and was not in good physical health. He had severe diabetes and Pott's disease, a kind of tuberculous arthritis that affects the spine. He was in such bad shape that his right foot and leg had developed gangrene. Three different doctors in New York City examined him and recommended amputation. Being the devout Buddhist that he is, he consulted the Dalai Lama. To say that the Dalai Lama went out on a limb is an understatement. He told Phakyab Rinpoche not to amputate, despite the fact that the doctors had unanimously told him he would die if he didn't. Instead, he advised him to meditate. The Dalai Lama said to use his skills at Tsa Lung meditation, a practice that opens the chakras and energizes the physical and emotional bodies, to heal himself. Taking what most people would call a huge leap of faith, Phakyab Rinpoche began his practice. He spent nine months meditating before his leg began to show signs of healing. At ten months he could walk on it with a crutch. After a year, he was completely healed. He is now being studied by researchers at New York University because current medical intervention cannot cure gangrene once past a certain point in its progression, except by amputation. Phakyab Rinpoche and the Dalai Lama had no doubt, even when his wounds were oozing putrid liquid and his pain and swelling had gotten worse.

---

5 George Bernard Shaw quote. (n.d.). Retrieved from
http://www.brainyquote.com/quotes/quotes/g/georgebern101824.html

They both knew that he would heal himself and then teach others the value of the ancient tradition. Heal yourself, and then heal all those around you. Can you think of a more noble cause?

Marcus Aurelius once said, "Everything we hear is an opinion, not a fact. Everything we see is a perspective, not the truth."[6] It is important to remember this, especially when we are hearing information about health and illness. Kathy Sykes, Professor of Sciences and Society at the University of Bristol, describes science in this way:

> Many people today believe Science can reveal truth.
> Science is a useful tool but it is far from perfect:
> ...science is not about truth, but is about trying to get closer to the truth. This is important because, too often, people look to scientists as having the "truth." What we have is wrapped in uncertainties, caveats, and simplifications.[7]

Holding too tightly to our beliefs or the beliefs of others is a mistake. This is especially so if you regard them as truths, because this will limit your possibilities. Truth is a verified or indisputable fact, proposition, or principle. How many actual truths are out there? Perhaps some mathematical truths would qualify: the truth of your sex, age, or nationality. Truths exist outside the bounds of society, what is acceptable, or political correctness.

It is okay to believe strongly in your ideas, especially when they are based in past experience. If I plan to do a 50-mile bike ride, I will believe I can do it because I've accomplished this in the past. If I have an idea that exercise will help my pain because I've found this to be the case, it will be a good thing to continue this practice. But when you are on a path to healing it is important not to be swayed too strongly by the beliefs of others, no matter how reputable or highly regarded they are. Their beliefs are based on their experience, not yours. There are too many people who are driven first by making a name for themselves, by getting media attention, and the best way to do this is by being sensational.

---

[6] This quote is a paraphrase from Meditations, Marcus Aurelius' hallmark work. Refer to the following for more information: Talk:Marcus Aurelius. (n.d.).
Retrieved from http://en.wikiquote.org/wiki/Talk:Marcus_Aurelius
[7] Sykes, K. University of Bristol Encylopedia of Philosophy. "Science and Truth." 2007. 2 April 2007.

In the noisy world we live in, the squeaky wheel gets the grease. The voices that say the most outrageous things, zealously defend their ideas, yell the loudest, and scare people the most are the ones that are heard. Institutions have much invested in people believing their version of the truth; so much so that they will try to berate and vilify those who don't agree with them. This is true for all sides of the health debate. You can get on quackwatch.org and read about the dangers of colloidal silver, acupuncture, or saunas. On the other hand, visiting many alternative health sites will lead to dire warnings about the use of "toxic" drugs and the nefarious pharmaceutical industry. Where is the truth in all of this? Is there any truth at all? Or is it all hype? The truth is that we'll never really know. The truth is we will hear many conflicting ideas about how to achieve health and treat illness. Ultimately we choose whom to believe. The best way to navigate the immense amount of information available in the realm of health is to remember that even a triple blind study does not guarantee the truth, that the loudest voices are usually the ones with the biggest ego at stake, and that, like Tibetan Lama Phakyab Rinpoche, you can create a new truth with belief. Your health and your life are dependent upon developing truths for yourself and holding tightly to them with a light fist.

So when you hear a claim made, especially a provocative one that will influence the way you see your health or disease, it would behoove you to ask yourself some questions. Is this making me feel worse or better about my life? Does this put more fear or more hope into my heart? What does the person making these claims have to gain from them? What is the risk and benefit to me? Medical fraud and misconduct in research are not uncommon; fraudulent studies have been published in major journals such as the British Medical Journal and the Journal of the American Medical Association. Retraction of medical research papers is at an all-time high. Ghostwriting, hiring respected experts in the field as named authors to give the appearance of credibility, is another ethically shaky practice that permeates research, especially research sponsored by industries that use it to promote products. In the health industry anyone can say anything, using testimonials to legitimize their claims. There are many supplement companies that use the multi-level marketing structure to sell their products. I've always liked the idea; to me it seems to be a win-win situation because each person buying the product stands to gain if they sell the product to others. However, this sets up a unique situation for encouraging the placebo effect. If you have the ability to make money off a product by taking it and telling others how well it works, then I'd be surprised if there wasn't a huge boost in the numbers of people who swear by the use of the product and truly think it helps them. I'm not saying that scientific research should be disregarded in the quest for health, just that when it comes to your health and your life everything you hear or read should be questioned before owning it as belief. Above all, if you want to be healthy from the inside out you have to feel good, and this starts with what you choose to believe.

I'm someone who has had a progressive disease for more than forty years. According to the experts, my prognosis is one of disability, chronic pain, elevated risk of depression, and early death. These may be the facts, but I don't have to take them on as beliefs. If I did I would be experiencing the Nocebo effect, the opposite of the placebo, where negative consequences are generated by a pessimistic outlook or expectation. What I believe is that everything is temporary; today I may have pain and disability and I may have this for years, but there is always the possibility of improvement, even complete remission. Believing this makes me feel better; it makes me healthier.

> Do not believe in anything simply because you have heard it. Do not believe in anything simply because it is spoken and rumored by many. Do not believe in anything simply because it is found in your religious books. Do not believe in anything merely on the authority of your elders and teachers. Do not believe in traditions because they have been handed down for many generations. But after observation and analysis, when you find that anything agrees with reason and is conducive to the good and benefit of one and all, then accept and live up to it.

This quote is attributed to the Buddha; the irony is that he most likely never said it. Considering the content, whomever actually wrote it must have a sense of humor. Regardless of who I believe is the true author of these words is beside the point. The point for me is the last sentence: Is your belief conducive to the good for you and those around you? If so, it is one to hold onto. If not, let it go. The secret to a healthy life may just be as simple as this.

PURPOSE

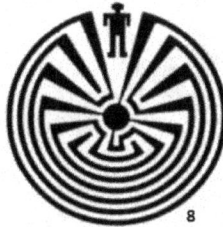

"Each Individual is Original Medicine.
Nowhere duplicated on the planet. Therefore
it is important to bring one's Creative Spirit,
Life Dream, or Purpose, to Earth."
- Angeles Arrien [9]

[8] "The Symbol of Life – Man in the Maze." The Symbol of Life – Man in the Maze. Symbols.com, n.d. Web. 28 May 2015.
[9] Arrien, A. (1995). Angeles Arrien essay: The Fourfold Way. Retrieved from http://www.spiritsound.com/arrien.html

What is the purpose of a life? Where does meaning come from? These are questions that most of us ask eventually. A life lived on purpose, consciously, looks a lot different than one that is lived on autopilot. It is the result of self-reflection, perseverance, and a commitment to your vision. It can come with grand ideas or simple truths; it can be challenging. Purpose is an inner commitment to living our truth.

There is no better catalyst in the search for meaning and purpose than illness. Illness strips away many of the roles and qualities that you once thought defined you. You can quickly move from feeling in control to feeling that life is spiraling away from you at warp speed. Suddenly you are no longer able to move through your day blissfully unaware of how tenuous your life and your health is. Illness can be savage; it can pound at you with a relentlessness that eventually brings you to your knees. Once you're on your knees you find that there aren't answers to be found there either and eventually you are on your back internally screaming for mercy. This is when you have to listen closely for a voice deep inside. It will tell you this: within the intensity of the experience of illness is an opportunity to discover who you really are and to begin to live in a way that reflects this. Your true meaning and purpose reside in the eye of the storm of your illness.

Since the advent of modern medicine in the 1800s, the way people perceive disease has changed. Scientists including Pasteur, Koch, Ehrlich, and Semmelweis proved relationships between germs and disease and this revolutionized the paradigm through which the lens of disease was seen. Disease was no longer explained holistically; instead there had to be an uninvited invader at the root of all illnesses. Treatment became a war, us against the germs. And since human beings seem to like a good fight, the singular focus of medicine has moved into combating disease at all costs.

The experience of disease isn't so simple. In modern society a person who is diagnosed with a disease inadvertently becomes a battleground. The doctors are the generals leading the crusade against the invisible invader of disease. Our symptoms are both the instigator of war and the body count. We are brainwashed into thinking that there is a right and wrong way to fight, that like Ghengis Khan leading the Mongols into battle our doctor has the perfect way to lead us into victory over disease. Each time we visit our doctor we trust that he has the correct strategy to find the right answers and the weapons to win the war. We look at the information the doctor has gathered through stealth spy-craft and physical intimidation, then watch as he comes up with a plan to win our unique war. Very soon, however, we realize that our doctor isn't Genghis Khan; he is the Wizard of Oz.

Illness, especially chronic illness, isn't a war. It is a journey. It begins with a physical crisis that soon becomes an emotional, mental, and spiritual quest for understanding. We begin by trying to understand what happened to create the disease, attempting to place blame. Then we move onto trying to figure out what to do to get rid of it. Hopefully, we finally begin to comprehend the true meaning of disease. Disease is an opportunity to live in the mystery while deeply understanding who we really are.

As much as I hate dichotomies, there is a clear division between those who live with disease and those who don't. Living in a body without disease affords you greater ease, more energy, and the ability to take certain things for granted. You can plan a trip without the added stress of wondering how your body will fare; you can exist for days with minimal sleep without intense repercussions, and you are more easily caught up in the cycle of busyness that is epidemic in the modern world. Living with disease, on the other hand, means that you don't take much for granted. You have a part-time job managing the symptoms that the disease produces. Conserving energy becomes paramount. You are the canary in the mine, the first to cough when the air isn't pure. Because your energy is precious, you learn not to waste it. When all of the busyness stops, when the distractions we so easily surround ourselves with get stripped away, what is left is simply you, pure and unadulterated.

There is a Cherokee teaching that speaks to purpose. It goes like this:

> One evening an elder Cherokee is teaching his grandson about a fight that goes on inside people. He said, "There is a battle that goes on inside us all. It is a terrible fight and it is between two wolves. One is evil – he is anger, envy, sorrow, regret, greed, arrogance, self-pity, guilt, resentment, inferiority, lies, false pride, superiority, and ego." He continued, "The other is good – he is joy, peace, love, hope, serenity, humility, kindness, benevolence,

empathy, generosity, truth, compassion, and faith. The same fight is going on inside you – and inside every other person, too." Grandson thought about it for a minute and then asked his grandfather, "Which wolf will win?" Grandfather replied, "The one you feed."

A person living with purpose is always feeding the second wolf. Purpose doesn't feed the ego because it isn't something you can rationalize or control. It isn't a choice; it is a calling. The only choice is whether you will listen and honor the purpose that you have been given. Purpose will eventually bring peace, but this doesn't mean a purposeful life is easy. More often, living a life on purpose means you walk down a road that might be a little scary, less settled, planned out, and easy to explain. It is a primal need, one that comes from an inherent yearning to become a whole person.

Purpose can also change as you grow. I think we all have more than one purpose. There is the purpose that you came here with, the reason for your life. Then there are the purposes that serve a time in your life, such as being a parent, writing a book, being a mentor to someone, or being present with someone who is at the end of their life.

"In the center of your own soul choose what you want to become, to accomplish ... Stick to it, never doubt. Say many times a day, 'I am that thing.'" –Ernest Holmes[10]

How do you discover your true purpose? First, you need to slow down long enough to listen. If you feel that your purpose is elusive you are moving too fast; often a purpose is found in plain sight. It is what brings you the most joy; it is what makes you feel the most alive and comfortable in your skin. It is where you find passion, excitement, and hope; it is what keeps you alive. It is where you are free. A wise person lives their purpose because it is the only way to become wise.

Recently I asked my friends and family the question, "If you had to answer the question 'what is the purpose through which

[10] Creative Mind and Success by Ernest Holmes - Read the Complete Text for free at NewThoughtLibrary.com. (n.d.). Retrieved from http://newthoughtlibrary.com/holmesErnest/CreativeMindAndSuccess/cmas_032.htm

you live your life right now what would you say?'" Here are some of the answers I got:

> "To learn my lessons of life: Humility, Humbleness, Self-worth, Strength, Compassion, Kindness, Grace, Truth = Wisdom."

> "Force of good"

> "To give a hand to whoever needs a hand. To find peace for myself and others. To find my purpose."

> "To heal my disease so that others will know that it can be done. To reflect back to others their true beauty so they can love themselves. To love and be loved. To help people help themselves."

The last answer was my own. My answer contains more than one pure purpose, but each complements the rest. By loving I will reflect to others their beauty and help them to help themselves. Practicing self-love is the only way to heal my disease, and by doing this I can teach others how to love themselves. When you find yourself having more than one purpose, there will be a thread that runs through them all. This is because, when you honor the purpose you came here with, your whole life reflects this.

How about the answer, "To find my purpose"? That is an interesting one, and very honest. Sometimes purpose can become elusive, and the search becomes the purpose. The search for purpose can lead to unexpected places. When I think of someone searching for their purpose I think of the book, *Eat, Pray, Love: One Woman's Search For Everything Across Italy, India, and Indonesia, by Elizabeth Gilbert*. If you haven't heard of this book, it is the story of a woman's search for herself. In the beginning of the book, Ms. Gilbert finds herself reeling from a divorce and in an unsatisfying rebound relationship. In order to fully disengage herself from her ex-husband, she gives him most of her money and possessions. As a successful writer, she is able to land an advance from her publisher for a memoir and she embarks upon a year-long journey. She decides to spend four months in Italy, eating and learning to enjoy life again. Then she goes to India, where she spends three months at an Ashram learning to meditate and get in touch with her spiritual side. Finally, she travels to Bali, reacquainting herself with a medicine man she had met during her last visit there, looking for the balance between enjoying life and living spiritually. What she eventually found in Bali was love and a true soul mate.

"'Tis better to live your own life imperfectly than to imitate someone else's perfectly." –Elizabeth Gilbert[11]

In the beginning of the book, Ms. Gilbert's life was lacking meaning or purpose. She had lost her joy. In deciding to take a year to search she did the most courageous and risky thing she could think of, somehow knowing that this was the right path. Her comfort zone was no longer comfortable, and she knew that she had to physically leave everything behind in order to find what was important. In the end, she found happiness. Her purpose was to live in this happiness and to share it with others. Her book has inspired countless people to do the same for themselves.

Not everyone has to travel to exotic locations in order to find their purpose. But, if finding purpose is your purpose right now, it is important to live each day with an open heart and mind. Ask to be shown, and open your eyes and ears to the answers that come. See everything that happens to you and the way you respond as clues. Soon, you will find that your purpose will come to you.

What if you're not sure whether you are living on purpose? Here are some clues; people who aren't living their purpose feel lingering dissatisfaction, an absence of peace, unfulfilled. Their life may look successful in a conventional sense, but it is reflective of decisions that were made to please others or some internal expectation of what they think they "should" be doing instead of who they really are. They are usually very busy and often feel frazzled. Victor Frankl, a psychiatrist who lived through the holocaust, and the author of the famous book *Man's Search For Meaning*, theorized that much of the modern angst that comes in the form of anxiety, depression, neurosis, and obsessive-compulsive disorder is caused by a lack of meaning and purpose. By finding meaning, one begins to live in service to a force greater than oneself. In doing so, one can transcend the ego and its investments in self-interest. He developed a

[11] "Tis' better to live your own life imperfectly than to imitate someone else's perfectly." – Elizabeth Gilbert. (n.d.). Retrieved from http://wise-quotes.net/10flq/

unique form of psychotherapy, which continues to be highly regarded, called Logotherapy. Logotherapy has three basic tenants.

- **Freedom of Will:** This is the ability to choose how to respond to any situation. With this comes the responsibility we have for our choices, our actions, and decisions.

- **Will to Meaning:** This is our primary motivation in life: the desire to find meaning and purpose. The will to meaning is essential for our health and survival and enables us to survive unimaginable sufferings, to persist in pursuing our dreams. The horrors that Frankl endured and witnessed during the Holocaust were a stark demonstration of this. In his book he described how he was arrested and taken to a concentration camp. He was newly married and was working on a new psychological theory. Before he was led away by the Germans he quickly sewed his manuscript into the lining of his coat. It was his life's work, his purpose at the time. Although he lost his coat soon after arriving at the camp he didn't give up. He continued his work during his imprisonment, observing the guards and prisoners and reconstructing the manuscript he had lost on stolen pieces of paper. Frankl witnessed time and again other prisoners who heard of the death of loved ones, or had their own meaning seemingly destroyed by their circumstances and died the next day. The will to meaning is also what enables people living with chronic pain, or severe disabilities, to keep going even when their situation is dire. Think of Christopher Reeves, Superman one day and a quadriplegic the next. Without his burning desire to walk again he wouldn't have lived as long as he did. Even though he never reached his goal, he inspired everyone who knew him and lived life to the fullest every day he had. His purpose and meaning propelled his physical body and enabled him to move beyond the limits that had been forecasted by his doctors and caregivers when his injury first occurred.

- **Meaning of Life:** This is the idea that meaning can be found even in the most miserable and seemingly intolerable of circumstances. The word Logos means both spirit and meaning. To Frankl, the spiritual dimension of life is the source of true purpose and meaning, which is why a person can endure most anything if they are living with meaning. As Friedrich Nietzsche famously said, "He who has a why to live for can bear almost any how." The spirit is much stronger than the human body and allows each person to tune into their "ultimate meaning." Frankl said, "The meaning of our existence is not invented by ourselves, but rather detected." Like the Buddhist First Noble Truth, Frankl believed that suffering is inevitable, and by tuning into the meaning of suffering one can find their path to a meaningful life.

Logotherapy describes the human spirit as the healthy core in each of us that can never be weakened. It can be blocked, especially with psychological illness, but it always remains intact despite what is happening in the body. The human spirit is the source of our hope, our creativity, our purpose and our meaning. It is our responsibility to discover our special purpose and to create a life that reflects this.

Once you've discovered your purpose you may want to write a personal mission statement. A mission statement provides clarity and helps you to frame your life. It reminds you of your purpose and tells you how to live. It has been described as a postcard of your life's journey. Your statement will tell you what you want to do and how you want to be of service. It will get to the core of who you are and provide you with guidance when making life decisions. A personal mission statement will help you to make good decisions and avoid getting off track. Instead you will be motivated by your purpose, by the essence of who you are.

Purpose and healing are intricately connected. To fully heal, you must move into your suffering instead of avoiding or numbing it. This takes courage, and the ability to withstand judgment and lack of understanding from those around you. Choosing to stand in your pain instead of trying to remove it will mean that sometimes you will be standing alone. As I said early in this chapter, modern medicine has brainwashed us into thinking that eradication of symptoms equal eradication of disease. In fact, subduing symptoms only serves to move the disease deeper, to entrench it and make it more difficult to access the real source of the illness. The symptoms we experience provide us with clues; they are one of the ways our body tells us we are out of balance. The suffering we endure is the catalyst for finding meaning, reaching deep into our spirit, and honoring our innate gifts. Without the suffering our gifts may remain hidden because we won't know how strong we are. Sometimes you just have to stand still, hold on tight, and ask for guidance.

"...the endurance of darkness is preparation for great light."
-St. John of the Cross[12]

Standing alone, determined to continue, finally surrendering, and asking for any and all assistance that may be available from your higher power is the bravest thing you will ever do. Not letting go of your meaning, and fully embracing your purpose in the midst of extreme suffering and lack of assurance from the outside world that all is okay, is true courage. Feeling the fear and doing it anyway will propel you to inner heights greater than you've ever imagined and allow you to be free.

There is an eye in the storm of your illness. When you find it never let go. It will lead you to your purpose. It will hold your hand when times get tough. And it will show you how to live. Commit to this wisdom and know that, as St. Theresa of Avila said, pain is never permanent. Behind the pain is healing. In order to heal you must feel. Feel the pain and find the meaning. You will never regret that you did.

[12] Dark Night of the Soul. (n.d.). Retrieved from http://www.spiritbride.org/A/spiritbride/dark_night.htm

MAVERICK

决心

"When I'm good, I'm very good. But when I'm bad I'm better."

-Mae West[13]

---

[13] Mae West quote. (n.d.).
Retrieved from http://www.brainyquote.com/quotes/quotes/m/maewest137976.html

All of the patients of the world, especially those who live with a chronic disease, have been fed a bunch of bologna. We've been told that to be a good patient we have to be compliant, take medication as prescribed, listen well to our doctor, and trust that our health care provider has our best interest at heart. The truth is that genuinely healthy people are mavericks. A maverick is someone who resists adhering to group decisions, and is independent in thought and action. Being a maverick means that when it comes to your health and your life, as George Bush so famously said, YOU are the decider. Your doctor is a highly educated, very well paid consultant who can advise you, but you are the true expert. As the expert, you always get to choose what is best for your health and your life.

Many people dealing with chronic illness have a story like this. At one point in my life the rheumatoid arthritis was so severe that my knees looked like they had grapefruits shoved inside the joints. I could barely move them and every movement was excruciating. When they weren't moving they were throbbing. So I went to a doctor who proceeded to aspirate my knees. Having a joint aspirated is not fun. Basically the doctor numbs the skin surface with lidocaine, pulls out a needle big enough for a horse, and sticks it in your joint space. Then he (or she) sucks up the fluid, which in a swollen joint looks like motor oil. All the while you are gritting your teeth and trying not to yelp. Afterwards they inject a steroid and you walk out with a somewhat normal-looking joint. Of course, like most medical treatments, this is a band-aide, not a cure, so four weeks later my knees were back where they started. Not that I'm complaining about the four weeks of relief, but I wasn't exactly looking forward to another horse needle either. I went round and round for a good six months having one or both knees injected until one day I knew it was time to stop putting the steroid in after the aspiration. There is a risk of joint damage if you do steroid injections more than once every three months and I was getting them monthly. I also noticed that when I went to a doctor who only injected one knee with steroid but aspirated both, the swelling came back at the same rate.

This was when I went to a new doctor, closer to home. She looked at my medical record and said that it would be a good idea to aspirate again. In walked the nurse with four needles, two horse needles and two that contained steroid. I told my doctor that I agreed with the aspiration idea, but didn't want the steroid. She looked at me incredulously and said that she had to do both at the same time. I explained the reaction I'd had when one knee didn't get the steroid and she didn't believe me. "That's just not possible, the steroid is an anti-inflammatory!" she told me sternly. I considered my situation. Here I was lying on the exam table with two extremely swollen and painful knees and here was my doctor, standing over me with a horse needle in her hand, about to stab me. She looked like she wanted to stab me, too, which was quite a shame, because until I had the audacity to direct my own care we had been very friendly. At the time I hadn't yet learned how to be a true maverick, so I relented. I was too scared of my angry doctor and her huge needles.

As I said, most people have been bullied in the doctor's office at some point. Bully may be a strong word, but then what else can you call someone wielding their power to make you do something you don't want to do? I always wonder why it is so threatening for doctors to have their judgment questioned. Do they really have such large egos? Or is it the opposite, that questioning them shatters the belief in themselves that they do have? How, in the autocratic environment of medicine, is one supposed to find healing?

When you are a patient it doesn't matter if you are a CEO of a Fortune 500 company or the guy who sweeps the streets, you will be humbled. Your time will no longer be valuable, your modesty will be a thing of the past, and you are almost guaranteed to encounter at least one health care professional whose emotional quotient is severely lacking. I have been on one side or the other of the treatment table for most of my life, and throughout my career as an occupational therapist I've often found myself in the role of patient advocate because so many people that I've treated over the years are lost souls. They've been told that they have a chronic, unremitting, and often painful disease, and then they are told to take their medicine and come back in a month. People who choose not to undergo standard treatment are ridiculed and ostracized. If you ask too many questions while in a hospital you're considered a pain in the butt and called a GOMER (get out of my emergency room). This was true in the seventies when the term was first coined, and sadly, not much has changed. Compassionate care is still something the medical profession has to talk about, meaning that it isn't already inherent the system as it should be. Shouldn't compassionate care, like a mother's love, be assumed? One would think.

"No man was ever great by imitation." –Samuel Johnson[14]

The millions of patients who are lost souls have become that way because they have allowed someone else to take their power away. They've willingly given over the health of their bodies to someone else. Once a patient is put into the hands of medicine, that patient will be thereafter guided only by logic and reason. Reason has its place, but healing is beyond reason. Healing happens when you stop being so damn logical and you start paying attention to the inner guidance that is always there. This guidance may seem untenable; that is when the maverick in you must come out.

My inner guidance has led me to places that sometimes surprise me and can be hard to explain. At times, even in the face of pain and swelling, I've decided to stop taking medication. Logically, this seems like a bad time to abstain, but inside I know that my body needs a rest. When I haven't given myself this rest, eventually my body becomes so hypersensitive that it begins to reject every medicine I try and over time I get sicker and sicker. On the other hand, I've entered medical trials that aren't time tested but I have a good feeling will help and they do. I also know that exercise is good for me and sometimes have chosen to push my body harder than those around me think is prudent. I always feel better afterwards. I've quit jobs that on the surface seem like good choices, but give me the Sunday blues. That feeling is a sign that I've learned everything I need to from it and it's time to move on. The decision is usually hard, but not once have I looked back.

All of us have qualities that can be our greatest strength or our largest obstacle depending upon how they are used. The key to being an effective maverick is to use your personal strengths to their best advantage. For me this means that I don't let my willpower turn into stubbornness, I don't let my high pain tolerance turn into stoicism, I don't let my perseverance turn into a useless waste of energy, and I don't let my happy nature turn into denial.

---

[14] "The Rambler" (1751) by Samuel Johnson; No. 154, September 7, 1751.

"Decide if you're a Tigger or an Eeyore." –Randy Pausch[15]

The Last Lecture is a best-selling book by Randy Pausch, a professor of computer science, human-computer interaction, and design at Carnegie-Mellon University. It is based on a lecture that Pausch delivered on September 18, 2007, entitled *"Really Achieving Your Childhood Dreams."* Professor Pausch was asked to give a lecture as part of an ongoing series where top academics were asked to contemplate what matters most to them, then give a talk imparting their wisdom as if it were the last lecture they would ever give. Ironically, one month before he was asked to be a part of the series Pausch was told that the pancreatic cancer he had been battling had spread. He had a terminal diagnosis with a prognosis of three to six months. The fact that this was going to really be, potentially, his last lecture gave Professor Pausch a unique opportunity, and he decided to talk about how to achieve your childhood dreams. In the book, he talks about the dreams he had as a kid including: play in the NFL, experience zero gravity, and work at Disney World developing new attractions. He talked about how each of his dreams was realized and about how the one that wasn't, playing in the NFL, may have been the dream that shaped him the most. Reading the book and hearing the lecture made me think about my own childhood dreams and something my good friend Ellen is fond of saying: *You are never too old to have a happy childhood!*

When I was in grade school I would spend my lunch hour writing stories. When I wasn't doing this I was writing plays that I'd direct and act in with my group of friends. I had a dream of being a child actor, starring in one movie, and then going back to "real life." This dream never came to fruition, partly because I decided not to join the acting club. I thought our acting teacher was mean and I didn't like how she treated some of the other kids, so in solidarity I abstained. Thinking about this, something else Randy Pausch talked about came to mind. Instead of bemoaning the fact that I never had my fifteen minutes of fame, I know that it's never too late to fulfill a dream. It's never too late to step into your own shoes and pursue the thing or things that make you happy. My dream of acting is fulfilled every time I step in front of a room of people and am able to inspire them, to give them hope. And my

15 Randy Pausch. (n.d.). Retrieved from http://en.wikiquote.org/wiki/Randy_Pausch

writing, which began in grade school and then went into hibernation for three decades, re-emerged when my disease prevented me from working. Life's twists and turns can lead to funny places; even though you can't direct the wind, you can move the sails. Remembering who you truly are, and deciding that you will let this guide you, will always lead to a surprising, fulfilling, and healthy life.

Albert Einstein, one of the most famous mavericks of all time, knew this. He was often described as impudent and although at times he did let this quality slip into casual disrespect, more often his impudence was reflected by boldness, the ability to draw outside the lines. He was always championing independent thought over punditry. If he was alive today I'm guessing that he'd be shaking his head so much at our current politics that he'd have a constant headache. Here are some more of my favorite Einstein quotes that reflect his attitude:

> *"Great spirits have always found violent opposition from mediocrities. The latter cannot understand it when a man does not thoughtlessly submit to hereditary prejudices but honestly and courageously uses his intelligence."*

> *"The important thing is not to stop questioning. Curiosity has its own reason for existing."*

> *"I am neither especially clever nor especially gifted. I am only very, very curious."*[16]

Jane Goodall is another one of my heroes. At first glance, few people would characterize her as a maverick, but in her own quiet way she is the master. As a child she loved animals, especially treasuring a stuffed chimpanzee she named Jubilee. This love eventually brought her to live in Kenya where she met Louis Leakey, a famous archeologist interested in how primates could teach us about early humans. With no formal degree, she became the first of "Leakey's angels," traveling with her mother to Tanzania to study Chimpanzees. It didn't take her long to shake the foundation of the scientific doctrine at the time. Instead of maintaining the appearance of objectivity, which is so prized by those who call themselves scientists, she developed relationships with her subjects. The first paper she

---

[16] Albert Einstein Site Online. (2012, January 8). Retrieved from http://www.alberteinsteinsite.com/quotes/einsteinquotes.html

gave outlining her findings was ridiculed. The language was too flowery, too familiar, and she actually had the audacity to name each chimp instead of numbering them, going against conventional practice. Jane ended up eventually blowing her critics out of the water through her astounding findings. She observed tool use, empathy and evil, life-long love, and systematic hunting. Chimps play, tease, and care for their ill, but also kill and torture one another. Jane's lack of formal training (which she made up for later by earning her doctorate in ethology) allowed her to see things no one else had. She was able to forever change the way the way we view apes and animals in general.

My favorite Jane Goodall story is this one. Medical research on chimpanzees is barbaric and the results to date have been questionable. Understandably, Jane was horrified by the practice and wanted it to end. Instead of becoming indignant and irate, as most people would, she decided to talk some sense into the head of one of the biggest medical research companies in the U.S. It took awhile, but she was able to eventually arrange a meeting, and during this meeting she carefully described what she had learned during her years living with chimps in Tanzania. The result of the meeting was close to miraculous. All medical research on chimpanzees at this company was stopped. One may criticize this decision, stating that someday, some disease may be eradicated through experimentation on chimpanzees, but Jane's thoughtful nature has been able to weather any storm of criticism that ensues as a result of her actions. Here are some of my favorite quotes from Jane Goodall:

> *"Change happens by listening and then starting a dialogue with the people who are doing something you don't believe is right."*

> *"Only if we understand can we care. Only if we care will we help. Only if we help shall we be saved."*

> *"The greatest danger to our future is apathy."*

> *"We have a choice to use the gift of our lives to make the world a better place."*[17]

---

[17] "Jane's Favorites!" The Jane Goodall Foundation. N.p., n.d. Web. 28 May 2015.

Sometimes in life there is a pivotal moment that forever changes you. I'll never forget the moment I realized that in order for me to survive I needed to become a maverick. While I had been working in a rehabilitation floor of a hospital I met a woman named Carol. Before seeing a patient, a therapist always reviews their medical chart. I was sitting at the nurses' station reading through Carol's medical record and I could feel my heart sink. Listed under her history were about ten diseases, any one of which would be gut-wrenching. Osteoporosis, diabetes, obesity, lupus, rheumatoid arthritis, osteoarthritis, and myasthenia gravis were all on the list. She was in the hospital because she had just undergone a knee replacement. So I steeled myself for a sad case and walked into her room. One thing I'd learned over the years was that you could work with a completely healthy patient who broke his wrist and you'd think from his reaction that the apocalypse had arrived. Or, you could see someone in dire straits, whose situation makes you want to cry and you'd end up laughing, happier than you'd felt in days, with a new outlook on life. Carol was an example of the latter.

Meeting Carol was like taking a breath of fresh air standing on top of a beautiful Swiss peak. She was the epitome of kindness, inner beauty, and had an attitude that makes us all look like pitiful whiners. I worked with her for a week, and ended up befriending her and her husband Max. Over the five years that I knew her I felt extremely grateful to have her in my life and learned much about the axiom, "attitude is everything." We shared many laughs and as two people living with daily pain, also a deep understanding of each other that transcended words. She cracked me up. One day she called me and said, "KAT! I found a way to sleep through the night! My son buys some of that marijuana that people smoke and my husband brews it into a tea. I drink the tea and my restless legs have stopped waking me up at all hours!" She laughed gleefully and said, "Now don't you tell!" Carol was a nice Christian woman.

I felt so proud of her. No one but those of us who have lived through prolonged bouts of sleeplessness will ever know just how horrifying this is. It is torture to the Nth degree and something you would never wish on a friend. Carol suffered every day, and the last thing she needed was for her suffering to extend into the night. Yet for years her myasthenia gravis had caused her muscles to randomly clench all night long.

Carol had been a "good patient" all her life. She carefully took the large dose of steroids that her doctors prescribed for many years. This contributed to three more diagnoses: obesity, diabetes, and osteoporosis. She politely offered herself as a guinea pig when, time after time, her doctors probed into her brain, stuck needles into her muscles, and prescribed yet another new drug, often to combat a side effect of another drug they had previously prescribed. She never complained a bit when all of these procedures made her suffering worse. She was courteous and kind to a fault; I never told her that this kindness wasn't always returned. While she was in rehab she was the butt of endless jokes about her weight. The culprit was our fearless leader, the physiatrist (an MD) who was in charge of our hospital floor. In our weekly meeting he amused himself for at least five minutes making fun of various patients. When Carol was visiting us and spreading her unconditional love, he spinelessly joked about her behind her back. The fact that her weight was directly related to the steroids she had taken, not overindulgence, must have conveniently left his mind.

One day I was visiting Carol at her house and she was describing yet another procedure her new doctor was going to do on her and suddenly I thought, "I'm not going to end up this way." I had a sudden realization that Carol had gone too far down the rabbit hole of medicalization to ever come out. She had taken too many drugs, had too many invasive procedures, and been a guinea pig one too many times to ever recover. She would end up dying from her good faith. And she did, two years later, when her body finally gave out. She didn't make it to sixty. Carol's legacy continues to inspire me, but her greatest gift was that she made me a maverick. From then on if a doctor wanted me to do something I felt would do more harm than good, I said no. My body is my most precious resource, and I will never let someone else plunder it.

"Know the rules well, so you can break them effectively."
–His Holiness the 14th Dalai Lama XIV[18]

Ivan Illich, an Austrian philosopher and Roman Catholic priest, was called a "maverick social critic" of contemporary western culture. In his book *Medical Nemesis*, Illich sharply criticized many aspects of Western medicine and what he called the "medicalization" of Western culture. He talked about how society has waged a "campaign against pain," which leads to a

[18] Kell, B. (n.d.). Dalai Lama: 18 Rules of Living. Retrieved from http://www.huffingtonpost.com/billie-kell/dalai-lama-18-rules-of-li_b_2572518.html

"state of anesthesia." [19] Society is determined to wage war against disease; we have had a sustained war on cancer, drugs, AIDS; you name it, we have waged war on it. Books aimed at helping those with disease reflect this. In my own search for help with rheumatoid arthritis I inevitably see these words in the title: how to beat arthritis, conquer or fight pain, or battle disease.

This ultimately sets the stage for a battle against self, a disowning of the lessons involved in disease, and the numbing of any symptoms that are distasteful to us or those around us. Pain in particular is the leprosy of our time. Admit that you live with pain and immediately you will have to answer questions about how you are going to get rid of it. The idea that the pain may not be vanquished is deplorable and unacceptable. "No, really, you HAVE to see a doctor!" I'll hear when I actually admit to my pain. The look in my companion's eyes changes with this conversation, and thereafter the pain is an endless topic. I thought a lot about this long before I'd ever heard Ivan Illich's comments, and my conclusion was that modern society has succeeded in avoiding physical discomfort to such a degree that it has become starkly afraid of it. Most of us are able to eat when we are hungry, stay cool in summer and warm in winter, and pop a pill for most any ailment that comes our way. Pain has become the bogeyman. Ironically though, addiction to pain medication is the new epidemic. This war against pain is yet another useless war that drains our precious resources. Our collective revulsion of pain hasn't made it go away. Quite the opposite, it clings to us even more.

In my own life I know that when I fight the pain my body responds by finding another way to talk to me. Like a game of Whack-a Mole, the pain goes down but then some other symptom pops up. So instead of aiming for eradication, I've developed a deep personal relationship with the pain. This relationship between pain and I has been a rocky one. Sometimes I wonder if, like a drunken sailor who wakes up with a tattoo, my spirit took a vow with pain without my conscious consent. Maybe there is such a thing as karma, and if so I know I am getting rid of a whole bunch of it in this lifetime. Maybe you do choose what challenges you will face in life before you come here. If so, next time I'm definitely choosing a huge physical gift like an amazing voice that needs to be harnessed,

---

[19] Illich, I. (n.d.). Full text of "Medical Nemesis" Retrieved from
http://archive.org/stream/MedicalNemesis/MedicalNemesis_djvu.tx

or the ability to climb mountains, or my personal favorite, inventing the most graceful way to surf ever seen. Pain has a way of giving you a very creative imagination. It's one way to leave your body when it's no longer being much fun. Pain has been my greatest teacher and has made me wise in ways I never would have imagined without it. It humbles me every day, and allows me to laugh at myself because sometimes that is all you can do. So many of the blessings of my life have ironically come from the pain and if I hadn't chosen to be a maverick, if instead I had followed the whims of society, I never would have allowed these blessings to come into my life.

"People who have been through illness's dark passage can occasionally give us a glimpse not only of what it is like to become whole, but what it is to be fully human." [20]
–Mark Ian Barasch

Mark Ian Barasch is an award-winning writer, producer, and editor who has written three books on healing that he calls his "healing trilogy." After reading his first two books, *Remarkable Recovery* and *The Healing Path*, his third book, *A Soul Approach to Illness*, was nothing short of life altering for me. In his books he describes his experience with throat cancer. Before, during, and after he was guided in his dreams about the process he would go through. After having surgery and being declared cured, his healing process truly began. This led him to research stories of spontaneous remissions and investigating how healing happens. He said:

> This was no academic pursuit, but a survival exercise; a way to ride out the aftershocks of a catastrophe still rumbling through my life. I was oddly gratified to discover that many of those I spoke to had also undergone inward shiftings of tectonic magnitude. Their crisis of the flesh had become, as had mine, a dilemma of the spirit. [20]

His eloquent approach to understanding illness and healing gave him valuable insights that he shares with his readers. He discovered that most people who were able to heal from

[20] Barasch, M. I. (1994, March). A Psychology of the Miraculous. Retrieved from https://www.psychologytoday.com/articles/199403/psychology-the-miraculous

incurable illness did the opposite of what was expected of them. They stopped focusing on "getting back to normal" and began a voyage of self-discovery.

This is only accomplished when you stop listening to the voices of the outer world and begin to listen with full attention to what you know to be true.

Living with juvenile rheumatoid arthritis for 95% of my life has been a rollercoaster ride and the best spiritual training ground that exists for me here on earth. Every day I've woken up with pain as my unwanted sidekick. Like an annoying puppy it jumps on me, yaps, and in general doesn't leave me alone. It is always changeable, so much so that it literally took me thirty-five years to realize that I have chronic pain. I'm not kidding. As an occupational therapist, most of my clients have pain-related issues and when I'd work with them I'd always think, "How tough that poor person's life is," putting them in a separate category from myself. When I finally woke up to my reality it amused me more than anything. I still prefer to think of my pain as a series of acute episodes rather than one never-ending fate that I endure. This trick of the mind enables me to stay in the moment and to experience life dynamically.

The experience of illness is a solo endeavor. Suffering isolates a person like nothing else. To others it is an intellectual exercise but for the person suffering it is all-consuming and beyond words. Illness can constrict your life to the point that you feel you are being suffocated and then just when there is no fight left in you, you are catapulted into relief. From the outside this relief looks like getting back to normal, but for the sufferer there is a deep understanding that life will never be the same again. You wait with bated breath until the next onslaught begins and when it does you tell yourself, "Here we go again." Most of my life I've had a recurring dream of being stalked by a sadistic killer that is only interested in killing me. I'll be surrounded by loved ones who are confused about my self-concern, disinterested in any defensive measures against my Monster, and as I try to hard to avoid my fate I feel dread in the knowledge that my actions are for naught, eventually I will get caught. This dread follows me in my waking life as well, part of the shadow side I've come to acknowledge.

Illness causes muteness on many subjects as well. When you know that by admitting to pain you will be left out, you just stop talking about it. For the many people free from chronic pain there is little understanding of the level of pain one can actually endure. Therefore the idea that a person would actually choose a painful experience is horrifying. "You push yourself too hard!!" I've heard time and again from well-meaning people. "What else can I do?" I wonder. "If I'm going to be in pain anyway, why not live the life I want?" I decided long ago that pain will never dictate who I am. Behind the brave face that I see on many people with cancer, the same mask I've used time and again, is a soul-level understanding that this experience is for us alone. Trying to explain it not only diminishes the experience, it also requires using a language that those not ill just can't understand.

"Solitude sharpens awareness of small pleasures otherwise lost." –Kevin Patterson[21]

The isolation that illness creates doesn't have to be a prison. It can actually be a refuge, a place to remember the truth of who you are. Illness provides a unique lens, an added texture to life. It can cause you to question yourself often with, "Am I still glad I'm here?" and "Where do I find my joy?" Because there is no escaping illness and pain you aren't able, like most people, to distract yourself with busyness and endless activity. This will only serve to make your situation worse. You have to search inside for the peace that is always there. It is a deep, endless well that nurtures you if you are able to find it. It is only found by getting quiet and traveling below the level of your thoughts and physical sensations. It is there to remind you not to judge, that everything is always okay.

Most people have to make a choice to empty themselves enough to see this place by visiting a monastery, going on a retreat, fasting, or something else to take them out of their comfort zone. However, when you live with disease being in a comfort zone is an abstract concept, not a reality. It's easy to understand the First Noble Truth of Buddhism, that the suffering of birth, old age, illness, and death are unavoidable. You don't need to spend thousands of dollars traveling to India on your quest for wisdom; you only need to sit back and buckle your seatbelt for the rollercoaster ride of your life.

---

[21] Kevin Patterson quote. (n.d.). Retrieved from
http://www.brainyquote.com/quotes/quotes/k/kevinpatte193134.html

Living in the unknown breeds fear and anxiety, especially in our modern, rational society. Pain and disease stubbornly resist all attempts at rational understanding. One can live, as I did, for years in a state of anxious reactivity to uncertainty. You'll find that when you do this there will be people who happily jump on your fear with you. When you talk to them you'll end up feeling more entrenched in your uneasiness and disease. You'll slowly become a victim and this will seep into every aspect of your life – particularly your relationships with other people. Society will fully support this state of being because society appears to feed on fear.

Eventually, you'll discover the antidote to living in fear and anxiety: becoming conscious. Being conscious means that first you observe your reactions and the reactions of those around you. You begin to shift the focus from trying to figure out and fix your predicament to living each moment with grace. You do the best you can whenever the next obstacle appears and then you trust that it will be okay, because really it always is. You learn to lighten up. You live every day what you know to be true and tune out the noise outside you. You trust yourself. You honor your personal principles and live them unwaveringly. You make a choice to be the wolf, not the sheep. You become a maverick and discover the secrets of true health.

HONESTY

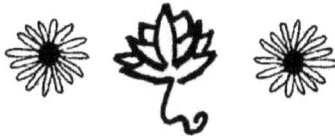

*"Honesty is the first chapter
in the book of wisdom."
– Thomas Jefferson[22]*

[22] Thomas Jefferson's Monticello. (n.d.). Retrieved from
http://www.monticello.org/site/jefferson/honesty-first-chapter-book-wisdom-quotation

We live in a post-truth society and it is ruining our health. Dishonesty is expensive. In 2011, 997 billion dollars was wasted on corporate fraud. It is epidemic in higher education; multiple studies have reported 50-70% of students in colleges and universities have admitted to cheating at least once. It takes the lives of young men and women in the military; since the age of the Roman Empire propaganda has been an effective tool for bringing countries into war. It is unavoidable; in the course of a day you will be lied to between 10-200 times. It is an evolutionary fact; the more intelligent the animal the more likely it is to be deceptive. Koko, a female Gorilla, who was taught to understand more than 1,000 signs in American Sign Language and 2,000 English words, was caught in a few whoppers. One day she blamed her pet cat for tearing the sink out of the wall. When confronted she signed, "Cat did it," and pointed to the innocent critter lying at her feet. It starts young; babies will cry if they are getting attention and stop if they are alone. By the age of three children understand that they can use language to tell you something that isn't true. We are all guilty of dishonesty. Statistics show that one in ten interactions between married people will involve a lie, and strangers will lie three times within ten minutes of meeting each other. Even if you're an outlier in the lying department I would venture a guess that you can remember a recent lie you've told. When I examine myself, I realize that even something seemingly innocent – like claiming, "No, I'm not cold" – counts.

Am I embellishing by talking about a "post-truth" society? Sadly no; at least a few books have been written about the topic. Farhad Majoo, the author of, *True Enough: Learning to Live in a Post-Fact Society*, says that people have cognitive traps, propensities for seeing things in a way that fits their ingrained beliefs. In his book he talks about how the growth of technology has created a unique environment for catering to peoples biases. Websites, youtube, facebook, even television and talk radio all help people to solidify their dogma and often muddle the truth.

This is an especially disheartening comment on society because it shows us just how disinterested in the truth people have become. The lies that we hear from our politicians are only spoken because they know that the benefit to them will outweigh the damage they will suffer if they are caught. If something is said enough times people will believe it as truth regardless, a fact that all politicians and marketing professionals are well aware of. A case in point: the rumor that

President Obama is a Muslim, patently false, has been repeated so often that more people are beginning to believe it is true. In 2009 one in ten Americans believed this false statement; in 2010 the number had grown to one in five. In society today it is hard to think of one profession that hasn't been tainted by dishonesty. Sports, law, medicine, politics, journalism, and even the clergy have all been mired in lies recently.

Dishonesty is not a modern invention. Since the advent of widespread print media there has been yellow journalism, or news that is more interested in sensationalism than facts. The term yellow journalism was first coined during the newspaper wars of William Randolph Hearst and Joseph Pulitzer II. The competition between their two papers was so fierce that each decided to sensationalize their stories. Hearst was instrumental in shaping American opinion, in particular regarding involvement in the Spanish/American War, and is famous for telling his star reporter in Cuba, Frederick Remington, "You furnish the pictures and I'll furnish the war."

"To believe in something, and not to live it, is dishonest."
–Mahatma Gandhi[23]

People are quick to criticize others for dishonest acts but most people will say that they are honest themselves. Dishonesty, though, can be a slippery slope that starts with justification. Many years ago as a new therapist I began my first job at a nursing home. In my first week on the job, I came face-to-face with decisions that can shape how you live your life.

I received a referral to see a patient who had just come home from the hospital. She was almost one-hundred years old and when I went into her room I met a tiny, frail woman who was ready to leave this world. At the time, nursing homes tended to be ruled by a few understood-yet-unspoken facts that greased the money wheels. Medicare paid the nursing home a lot more for a person receiving therapy. Anytime a resident of the nursing home went to the hospital for forty-eight or more hours they were eligible for therapy under Medicare part A, which paid much more than what the nursing home received for the daily care of a resident. This meant that there was great

23 Quotes and Meanings. (n.d.). Retrieved from
http://mahatmagandhiproject.weebly.com/quotes-and-meanings.html

incentive to get doctor orders for therapy anytime someone went to the hospital for any reason.

As a new therapist I was aware of these rules, but unaware of the implications until I walked into the room of my new patient. She was so obviously not appropriate for treatment. To be appropriate for therapy there has to be an expectation of improvement, and in good faith I could not see this potential in her. But there was also something else driving my decision; she did not want therapy. At almost one-hundred years old the last thing she wanted to spend her final days doing was arm exercises. I had to respect her wishes and my truth, so I screened her, talked to the nurses, and went on with my day.

That was not the end of the story, however. Later that afternoon I got a call from my boss. He was one of the partners of this small company and the man who had recruited me for the job. "Kat, I heard you let Mrs. Smith go today. I want to come and show you some ideas for her treatment."

He was using this as a teaching moment, but the lesson I learned was much different from the one he intended. As I watched him try to rouse Mrs. Smith from a deep sleep, my heart sank. "Well, I think she'd be a great candidate for a hand splint. See how her wrist has become contracted?" He pointed to her left hand, which was, in actual fact, a bit contracted. (This means that it has become so stiff that it no longer moves in its full range of motion.) He wanted me to order a splint for her and spend the next month attempting to get a few more degrees of range of motion in her non-dominant hand. Ostensibly, the reason for this was to provide her with the best care available. However, as someone who wore hand splints for most of my childhood I know how painful they are, especially when wearing them for a prolonged period of time on a contracted hand. I could imagine the pain and suffering Mrs. Smith would endure if I followed my boss's strong recommendation and I had to say no. I knew that by giving into him my slippery slope into therapeutic decisions based more on the bottom line than on what was best for my patients would begin. This job ended up teaching me many lessons about the danger of justification, and I finally left when I found myself falling prey to the justification morass.

At the time, my company had started a new incentive program for therapists. They offered each therapist profit sharing, which meant that for every patient we saw we would receive a percentage. Therapists all over the company were jumping at the chance, hiring a bunch of new aides, and bulking up their caseloads. The company began raking in the dough and I smelled a rat. Something told me that doubling the number of patients and maintaining quality of care was impossible, particularly if at least half of them were being seen by aides who didn't have a college degree, let alone a therapy license. I was finally pressured into joining this new program, telling myself that I would remain untouched by greed. Then the paychecks started flowing in. I was being paid more than I'd ever imagined. It felt good. I started to scheme about increasing my caseload. My paycheck rose. And then one day I woke up. I saw myself in a few years, sitting on a bunch of money, looking at my therapy gym filled with aides and uncomprehending patients. I saw myself becoming my boss. And I quit.

My boss was surprised and thought it was a gambit to ask for even more, so he started bargaining with me. When I turned him down I walked away feeling happier and freer than I'd ever felt in my life. I've never again made so much money in my life and I've never missed a penny.

"If you do not tell the truth about yourself you cannot tell it about other people." –Virginia Woolf[24]

Pamela Meyer, author of *Liespotting, Proven Techniques to Detect Deception*, says that lying is a cooperative act. It involves the liar, and the person who agrees to believe the lie. We become vulnerable to lies, and more willing to cooperate in a lie when we are attempting to connect "how we wish we were" with "who we really are." In her book, Ms. Meyer poses the question, "What are you hungry for?" Are you hungry for money, fame, prestige, respect, admiration, love, feeling desired? The answer will help you to understand where you are most vulnerable to lies. This leads one to a universal truth: You can only be as honest with those around you as you can be with yourself. This is a truth I realized long ago, and when I did it made me sad. Every time I'm lied to I see the person who is lying as someone who is disconnected from the truth of who they are. This is the enormous tragic personal cost of dishonesty and one that inevitably permeates outward, creating our post-truth society.

---

[24] Virginia Woolf quote. (n.d.). Retrieved from
http://www.brainyquote.com/quotes/quotes/v/virginiawo131850.html

When I think about personal dishonesty I can't help but wonder, "What is so scary about the truth? Why do we hide the truth from ourselves? What would happen if we all were brave enough to whisper the truth quietly to our private self?" If we could remember our truth, respect it enough not to be swayed by the lies we hear outside ourselves? If we listened to a truth stated by Marcus Aurelius so many years ago: "If it is not right, do not do it; if it is not true, do not say it." Maybe then, we would enter a post post-truth society.

If Pamela Meyer is right about our vulnerability to lies, the cure should be to stop being so hungry. The only way to do this is to bridge the gap between who you are and who you think you want to be. You have to begin to commit to living authentically and with compassion for yourself. If we can begin to take the search for truth more seriously than we do the need to be lied to life as we know it would begin to change. If we held ourselves accountable for the little and the big lies that we tell and choose to believe, the direction of our life would change. Even the little lies count.

> Truth or reality is avoided when it is painful. We can revise our maps (of life / reality) only when we have the discipline to overcome that pain. To have such discipline, we must be totally dedicated to truth. That is to say, we must always hold truth, as best we can determine it, to be more important, more vital to our self-interest, than our comfort. Conversely, we must always consider our personal discomfort relatively unimportant and, indeed, even welcome it in the service of the search for truth. Mental health is an ongoing process of dedication to reality at all costs.
> –M. Scott Peck[25]

I agree with Mr. Peck. The truth can hurt, especially when you turn the lens of truth onto yourself. It takes a really brave person to be committed to self-truth, and a strong person to change herself when the truths she discovers reveal that she has been inflicting harm on herself or others. The commitment to self-truth involves a lot of questioning, asking yourself why you believe what you do, why you say the things you do, why you've developed the habits you have, if you are truly happy,

---

[25] Peck, M. S. (2003). *The road less traveled: A new psychology of love, traditional values and spiritual growth* (p. 50). New York: Simon & Schuster.

what parts of your life are healthy, and where dysfunction has become ingrained.

Embracing the muddy waters of life while you dig for the truth of who you are will make the process easier. Or as my friend Ellen says, "Try to avoid blame and guilt, and instead, be disciplined yet gentle." As you become more thoughtful about your life and relationships, you will grow new eyes. They will help you to recognize when you are in a relationship or an interaction that feeds the unhealthy parts of yourself. This is when you can choose to stop feeding them. You really don't have to join the party, even if you have attended this party for most of your life. Change your reaction, tell the truth, and the other person will have to change; always remember that it takes two to tango. You also have the choice to move away and let others be. As the Dalai Lama says, "Silence is sometimes the best answer." And finally, sometimes self-truth is enough. If you make a poor decision or tell a lie, you can choose to be honest with yourself, take accountability, and try to do better the next time.

Three enemies to honesty are justification, ego, and rigid thinking. When you begin to hold yourself accountable to being honest, these insidious enemies will show up countless times every day. Justifications are nothing more than excuses, a way to give yourself a pass for actions that you know are wrong. You can justify nearly anything, and once you open your ears to these excuses the sound will quickly become deafening. Does recycling really take too much time, or are you just not that interested in taking the steps necessary to reduce waste? Are you too busy to exercise, or just unwilling to give up time in front of the television? Are you staying at a boring job because of the economy, or because if you found one more suited to your abilities you may have to work harder? Have you not left an unhealthy relationship because you're not sure whether he or she is the one, or because you do know but are afraid to be alone again? Did your jeans really shrink? The honest answers to these questions may not put you in the most flattering light, but sometimes the truth hurts. When you begin to question your justifications, you will come face to face with your shadow side; this is where the ego resides.

The ego exists to protect you, sometimes from the truth of who you are. It provides you with a strong sense of self, the "I" that you use to define yourself. It tells you what you like and don't like, what and who you believe, and what you will do or not do.

It builds you up in your mind and provides safeguards when your faith in your mental ideas begins to falter. The ego has an important purpose, helping you to survive, but in the modern world it has become bloated with overfeeding. As a good friend of mine has told me, "beware of the insidious ego."

If you haven't been humbled lately, you know your ego is in control. By inflating our idea of self, the ego creates a false sense of separateness, cutting us off from others, our spiritual life, nature, our responsibility, our destiny, and our true purpose. The truth will set you free; the ego keeps you in prison. It does this by causing us to resist change, which impedes personal growth, and also by closing our eyes to the truth. When we see something in ourselves that we don't like or want to think about, the ego jumps in and provides justifications, biases, or assumptions that lift the burden of facing hard truths. This may make you feel better temporarily, but in the long run this habit directly blocks healing. To avoid constant self-justification, you have to commit to self-truth.

Looking outside yourself it is easy to spot dogmatic speech: rigid doctrine spoken and held tightly by ego-driven pedants (pedagogues). These people answer every question with a speech that resembles a broken record, give every excuse in the book for remaining right where they are, and become patronizing and filled with ridicule when questioned. They appear to feel safe, secure, and better than, yet their cup runneth over with the lies they tell themselves. It's harder to recognize this person in yourself, but this recognition is imperative in a true quest for health. Looking in the mirror before you begin to point fingers at others is a brave and scary thing to do, which is why most people would rather hold fast to their misbeliefs and rationalizations.

Cultures are defined in large part by their language. In the Tibetan language there is no word for guilt; instead they talk about intelligent regret. Intelligent regret is the ability to replace guilt with accountability. People who practice intelligent regret will look back on their past and without judgment observe how their decisions have affected their life and the lives of those around them. They then ask themselves, "What can I learn from this? How can I handle a situation like this better in the future?" The wisdom gained from the answers to these questions increases a person's self-honesty. A person practicing intelligent regret can see with clearer eyes and tell themselves, "I will not act this way again; this behavior doesn't reflect who I am." If you practice intelligent regret, over time you will find that you say what you mean, mean what you say, and live what you believe or consciously choose not to. It increases humbleness and wisdom.

Compare intelligent regret to the habit of assigning guilt that most people have cultivated. With every circumstance that is seen as negative or hurtful someone has to be blamed. Apologies may be handed out, but usually behavior doesn't change. Hurt feelings build up and over time relationships deteriorate, sometimes to the point of no return. Without accountability, the person feeling hurt will become a victim, not realizing that they've chosen to: (a) listen to or be near the person hurting them; (b) believe the other's words at least a little, otherwise they wouldn't feel hurt or allow the other's actions to affect them, and (c) allow their thoughts or the other's actions to stay negative and ruin their day, week, month, year, or life. The person misbehaving can ramrod over everybody and blithely say, "I have no regrets!" When I hear someone say they have no regrets I cringe inside a little because I know they aren't promoting self-honesty. Instead they are getting really good at justifying bad behavior.

You'll find that when you stop assigning guilt, you'll experience less life drama. Most of the drama will happen as you hold yourself and sometimes others accountable for their actions. This is useful because it is part of growth, but as someone with increased awareness you will know that sustained life drama is a sign you are stuck in a negative pattern that you need to get out of. Learning to live with intelligent regret will halt patterns of hurt and plant seeds for a life filled with true compassion and love.

An honest effort towards true health begins with self-reflection about the unreasonable sides of your nature, the "magical thinker" that sets you up for disappointment and resentments. Unraveling the lies you've told yourself and clung to for so long takes time. Shedding the ideas and biases that aren't yours will allow you to grow, just like the snake who sheds its skin. You must commit to truth despite what those around you or the world at large is doing and refuse to stoop to the lowest common denominator when it comes to honesty. The only way to begin to change the flow of the river is to be the first rock that settles in where it belongs. Once this process is in motion, life may get shaky for awhile before finally, for the first time you can remember, it begins to feel right.

For more than half of my life my magical thinker refused to believe that my disease affected me at all. I pushed hard, did everything to prove how "healthy" I was, and never talked about the truth of my experience. The unrelenting pain and swollen joints were irritations to be subdued, not listened to. When the disease reared its ugly head to the point where hiding it from others was impossible I turned my anger and frustration inward, railing at myself. My ego-driven internal taskmaster placed blame at my feet. This doesn't sound like a very protective ego, but actually it was. By placing blame, my ego was protecting me from the scary truth that my disease did make me different, it did shape me to my core, and it wasn't going away no matter how much I refused to talk about it. Sometimes the truth of who you are doesn't look like who you want to be, but resisting this truth will do far more harm than boldly facing it. Finally facing the fact that the rheumatoid arthritis is a lifelong companion that makes me more vulnerable and physically weak in some ways is a hard pill to swallow, but it allows me to open the door to self-compassion, which is the greatest healer of all.

"I undertake the precept to refrain from incorrect speech."
–The Fourth Buddhist Precept[26]

The Fourth Buddhist precept of right speech is found in the Noble Eightfold Path. The Buddha carefully laid out the Eightfold Path for people who choose to follow the path of Buddhism, and like many Buddhist concepts it is multilayered and designed to be used in a lifetime of committed practice. What is helpful about this specific precept is that it provides a guide for a person who has decided to be serious in their quest for truth-seeking and truth-telling. The basic questions one must ask in this practice are: "Do my words help or harm? Do they promote good will or divisiveness?"

Obvious forms of speech to avoid include abusive speech, lying, and idle chatter. This may seem simple, but here is where the layers come in. Sometimes one will tell a lie without knowing one's statement is false and this may still be a sincere attempt at right speech. Then again, if you carelessly pronounce

---

[26] O'Brien, Barbara. "The Fourth Buddhist Precept, The Practice of Truthfulness." About Religion. About.com, n.d. Web.

something as the truth without making the effort at due diligence in checking it out first you would be breaking the precept.

Another facet of this precept is that if you tell a truth to someone that hurts them to hear but actually helps them, then you are practicing right speech. There is a difference between "hurtful" and "harmful" in this context. Hurtful may be right speech; harmful is never right speech.

"The words of the tongue should have three gatekeepers"
—Arab Proverb[27]

This ancient proverb has roots in the Sufi tradition, and is tied to the Buddhist Eightfold Path. It tells a person to ask three questions before speaking.

- Is this **True**?
- Is it **Kind**?
- Is it **Necessary**?

I've also heard of a fourth question sometimes added on, "Is this **Timely**?" These four questions crystallize the practice of honest speech. Sometimes the truth isn't kind, and the only reason to speak it is to boost one's ego. If your speech is coming solely from a place of self-concern it isn't necessary, regardless of its truth. How often do we find ourselves in conversations about other people that have no purpose other than to boost the speakers up in their own minds? Office banter can be the worst offender in this category. People spend much time monitoring the work of others instead of focusing on the task at hand – complaining about the bosses, or management, instead of problem-solving. In more than one of my jobs I had ineffective bosses, people who landed in management because of their longevity with the company rather than their leadership skills. Inevitably, people would complain about them to the point that I would begin to tune them out. Here is Marcus Aurelius:

> When you wake up in the morning, tell yourself: The people I deal with today will be meddling, ungrateful, arrogant, dishonest, jealous, and surly. They are like this because they can't tell good from evil. But I have

[27] Thought for the Day | Blue Mountain Center of Meditation & Nilgiri Press. (n.d.). Retrieved from http://www.easwaran.org/thoughts-for-the-day-quotes.html?thoughts=8%2F2

seen the beauty of good, and the ugliness of evil, and have recognized that the wrongdoer has a nature related to my own – not of the same blood or birth, but the same mind, and possessing a share of the divine. [28]

"Suffer hard words," the Buddha says, "as the elephant suffers arrows in battle. People are people, most of them ill-natured."[29] The Buddha was realistic in his assessment of the majority of people. He realized that living in the world a person will be surrounded by wrong speech, sometimes directed at you, sometimes elsewhere. What is a person to do in when this happens? You can get angry and chastise the offender, but that would be wrong because it wouldn't be helpful, and would only elicit an angry response. Or you can choose to continue to act in you integrity, and honor your commitment to right speech.

When I wrote my first book for people with rheumatoid arthritis I was a neophyte in the world of being an author. In doing my due diligence on promoting the book I was often amused, and sometimes dismayed, by what I was reading. I was counseled to make sweeping statements that would grab headlines, to become an expert by joining trade organizations and reading a few books, to create a simple plan that I could teach others so I could have my own niche. All of these actions would have garnered attention with little regard to the truth. There was no way I was going to heed this advice despite the fact that it was coming from the experts in the field because I held fast to my own truth: When it comes to healing, the true expert is the person who is being healed. Even someone who has lived with the same illness for 40 years can only provide options, give advice, and validate experience; they cannot tell another person what to do.

Committing to speak truth regardless of the sea of words that surround you is difficult but necessary on the path to health. Speaking only words that help, and never ones that harm, will not only make you feel better but will also ease the suffering of all those around you. When pondering this idea, I began to wonder if withholding information is a form of lying. I posed this question to a wise friend of mine and he said, "It depends on what information you are withholding. If you know someone needs to lose weight, you don't have to tell her. Most likely she

---

[28] Meditations. (n.d.). Retrieved from http://en.wikipedia.org/wiki/Meditations
[29] The Elephant. (2009, June 25). Retrieved from https://eddietwohawks.wordpress.com/2013/06/25/the-elephant-3/

already knows this. But if she asks you if she needs to lose weight, then you should tell her." I've thought about times that I've avoided saying something important because I knew the person I was speaking to would get angry or upset. Over the years this has put distance into my relationships, and when I decided to heal my life I knew I'd have to stop doing this. Now, when I have something difficult to say I put thought into how I will say it. I've come to find out that if you come from a place of true love and caring for the person you are talking to, the result of this will always be positive.

A few years ago my older brother was deathly ill. Being the tough guy that he is, it took awhile before the family woke up to the dire nature of his situation. He has a disease that affects his kidneys, and at that time his kidney function was abysmal. I was in another state, thousands of miles away, hearing facts over the phone. He was exhausted; work and sleep were all he had energy for. His blood pressure was high, and his doctor was on vacation. When asked, he told my Mom that he would go to the doctor in a few weeks, end of discussion. My Mom described his condition to me over the phone. She told me, "Your Dad says he's fine. Ned barks at me when I ask how he's doing, but all he does is lie on the couch and sleep." I told my Mom that she was going to have to be brave, and go tell my brother that he had to see a doctor ASAP. I said, "Just do it as soon as we get off the phone. I'll be praying for you." I knew I was asking a lot. Ned is 6'2" and can be very formidable.

My little Mom took a deep breath, marched into the family room, and practiced right speech. She spoke firmly but with love and told Ned she was going to take him to the hospital. My little brother met them there and wouldn't let the ER staff send him home until the test results came back. Good thing, too, because my brother was a heart attack waiting to happen. Right speech can be hard, but it saves lives.

Right speech is also tactful. It involves first remembering the Buddhist precept to only speak words that help, never harm. Without this intention speech quickly degrades into useless noise: reactive, emotional, and ineffective. The reason for speech is to communicate: information, analysis, advice, understanding, assistance, reassurance, emotion, and feeling, with the intent to receive feedback and/or validation. The best way to do this is by being clear about your intentions.

To effectively get your message across, clearly and honestly, always thinking "win-win," especially during important conversations. How many times have you said something and wanted to eat your words? Words said in haste or anger can do a lifetime of damage, especially to a child or loved one. The adage "Sticks and stones will break my bones but names will never hurt me" is just not true. Emotional abuse of anyone, especially a child, will systematically break down self-esteem. It will lead to feelings of anxiety, disconnection, shame, guilt, helplessness, and, over time, physical breakdown. Sadly, people who use harsh words on others are often just reflecting their own wounds. The words one says to others reflect the words one says to oneself. Children easily absorb the words of the adults around them, believing what the adults say. If a child observes adults who throw around harmful words, this child will forever be tainted by these words. How many things can you remember hearing as a child that you can't forget? How many things have you heard spoken by an intimate partner or loved one that you can't get out of your head? How many of these statements are actually true?

My good friend Leah is beautiful on the inside and out. I met her when I first moved to Salt Lake City and I saw her dog Max sitting next to her at a coffee shop. Max was so huge and adorable I had to pet him, and he led me to a lifetime friendship. Since that day Leah and I have spent days hiking, dreaming, and talking about our lives. A few months after I met her she started dating a new man and after a whirlwind romance she married him. The marriage had a very brief honeymoon period, and then quickly became less than idyllic. Her husband regularly commented negatively on her looks, her body, and her personality, despite the fact that Leah is a natural beauty; she'd be at home on the cover of Outside Magazine. She does not spend three hours applying makeup in the morning and she doesn't need to. Once married, though, I saw her change. She lost an unhealthy amount of weight, and began to be anxious about her looks. Her marriage only lasted a few years, but the words that she heard during this time echoed in her head much longer.

"Primum non nocere, First Do No Harm"
–from the Hippocratic Oath

If medical practitioners would take the fourth Buddhist Precept to heart when they recite the Hippocratic oath there would be a lot fewer ill people. There are numerous accounts of people dying shortly after being given a terminal diagnosis by their doctor, who later discovered that the diagnosis was incorrect. Of course, technically this is still right speech because the doctor believed the falsehood at the time. The problem I've always had is with the offhand comments I've heard over the years. "You have a disabling disease. You won't be able to do that again. People in your condition will eventually need a joint replacement. People don't recover from this. You're going to have to expect a lifetime of pain." Are any of these statements true, kind, and necessary?

Then there are the comments said behind a person's back. As a therapist, I've heard more of these than I ever care to remember. Comments by health-care practitioners about a person's weight, looks, or sensational statements about mental and emotional states are completely unnecessary and harmful even if the person isn't in the room. These comments taint the views of those who hear the comment and then later work with the person about whom the comments were made. This is a problem that permeates workplaces everywhere. Honest speech will never defame or denigrate another.

When you live with a chronic disease, honest speech about your condition can be difficult. A casual "How are you?" if answered honestly, can result in uncomfortable silences or pat responses. How does one honestly reveal the complexity of their situation, the extreme discomfort and uncertainty daily life can bring, the sadness and frustration that disease can cause? What has always worked best for me is the "need to know" test. If someone needs to know the information I will tell them, and if they really don't I will keep it to myself. I do this because I know that sometimes my truth can cause anxiety and worry in others, especially loved ones. It also can invite unwanted advice and unsolicited opinions. If I tell someone how much pain I'm in often he will feel that he needs to do something to alleviate it, or to tell me what I should do. If I get asked, "How are your knees today?" I'll answer without mentioning the fact that my elbows and ankles are hurting unless the person asking will be impacted in some way by that pain. This means much of my pain is unspoken. After forty years of living with pain, I've come to understand that this is the healthiest and most honest way I can respond to it.

I leave so much unspoken because the truth is that much of the experience of living with disease defies words. How can words describe the ungraspable nature of pain that makes it so subjective and changeable? Who is the captain that steers the ship of disease? How can you find him and plead your case? How do you explain the unexplainable? People who aren't saddled with the experience of chronic pain and disease will have to learn this truth some other way; life is a mystery, and learning to honor this truth instead of solve it saves a person much angst. I choose carefully those people who fully enter my world; these are the people who can respect the mystery without letting their ego butt up against it. This isolates me somewhat in my experience, but this is okay. The truth is that although we are all connected, we also all experience life alone, each in our unique bodies and minds.

Kiril Sokoloff, author of the book *Personal Transformation: An Executive's Story of Struggle and Spiritual Awakening.*, became deaf as an adult and throughout his book he talks about the isolation in his experience of being deaf:

> ...a professor of history is giving a lecture. She shows us a slide presentation of ancient art. The overhead light is on at the beginning of the presentation but after a few minutes her husband turns the lights off. Without lights, I can no longer comprehend the lecture, but the twenty people in the room see the intricate beauty of the slides more clearly. The dilemma? Do nothing, miss the lecture, enjoy the slide show, and be happy that everyone has a clear view of the beautiful, ancient art? Or to make a fuss and turn the lights back on? Of course, I choose to remain silent, as I have a thousand times, when people turn down the lights, turn up the music, take me to noisy restaurants, and talk at the same time, interrupting each other constantly.[30]

This description at first seems depressing and sad. It is a stark reminder of how easy it is to be completely alone in a room filled with people. When I read it my first reaction was to feel bad for Kiril, but at second glance I realized something else. In this interaction Kiril was being completely honest with himself, and in choosing not to speak up he was practicing true kindness. He was giving those around him a gift, knowing that most of the people in the room would never be aware of his offering, and his selfless act wouldn't have been possible if he

---

[30] Sokoloff, K. (2005). *Personal transformation: An executive's story of struggle and spiritual awakening.* New York: Crossroad Pub.

had spoken up. His thoughtful understanding of both himself and those around him stemmed from his ability to be honest without attaching any self-defeating emotions to the situation. He was demonstrating the actions of someone comfortable in his skin, with a frank understanding of his situation.

Sometimes not speaking can be the most honest and selfless thing you can do. Modern psychology places much emphasis on talking things out, speaking up and expressing emotions. If you have a problem, you have to discuss it with your loved ones and friends. If you have been abused or traumatized the healthy thing to do is to let it out, because keeping it inside will only serve to make it worse. The problem isn't with this idea; it is how people interpret it. Talking about your situation is healthy in the right context, but if you keep talking about your wounds you will stay wounded.

Wounds can teach us how to be honest with ourselves. When you hurt it becomes harder to fool yourself; your pain will always be there as a truth meter as you feel the consequences of your decisions and thoughts. For much of my life I fought this knowledge. The fear of living the life I was called to was so much stronger than the discomfort caused by living at odds with the truth of who I was. This continued until my body stopped being a nuisance to be handled and began to become a gorilla on my back, pounding me to the ground. I finally became so sick that I could no longer lie to myself. The lies took too much energy. Even the simple justifications about the choices I made sounded hollow to my ears. My ego surfaced and fought with my truth. It really wanted me to be "normal," by maintaining a "regular life," which included a professional job, a family, and stability. All the while my life was calling me in a different direction: simplicity, freedom, true connection, adventure, flexibility, love, leading by example, communion with spirit; this is where my heart was leading me. Truth eventually won and I began to follow my heart. Like Tim DeChristopher, who bid on 22,000 acres of federal land knowing he couldn't pay for it because he couldn't bring himself to let it go to corporations who were going to defile it, I jumped off the cliff and then I learned to fly.

Without knowing what I was going to do next I quit my job, left my boyfriend, stopped my medical regime, and moved away from my house. I moved back to the small town that had been calling me in my dreams. I began to write. People, opportunities, and experiences that showed me who I truly was began to show up. My body began to change, every so often showing me windows of health and a pain-free existence I'd only dreamed about. As these windows opened, my belief began to grow. The hopelessness that had always permeated my inner life gave way to hope.

I found that once you stop hiding from yourself your life will never again be boring. You will spend a lifetime learning and teaching others. You will have to make many brave choices, often alone, and then live with their consequences. You will need to begin a practice of self-honesty and right speech until honesty replaces self-deception as your natural state. There is no other path to true health; you must walk towards the truth of who you are, even knowing that living honestly may take a lifetime to achieve. It's important to get on this path, and it's important to keep trying.

EFFORT

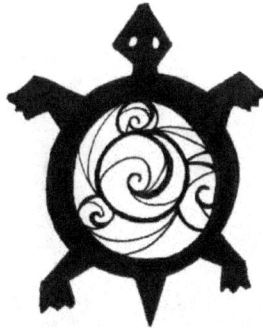

[31]

"What would life be if we had no courage to attempt anything?"

-Vincent Van Gogh[32]

---

[31] Turtle symbol created by Alexandra Albert
[32] Vincent Van Gogh quote. (n.d.). Retrieved from
http://www.brainyquote.com/quotes/quotes/v/vincentvan150781.html

Every so often throughout this book I'm going to do what I call a "Willieism" in honor of Willie Nelson. This man, I recently discovered, knows a thing or two. He also has a way of making big truths simple. Here is one I like a lot: *Beyond the basics of who you are, the rest is mostly creative use of adjectives.*[33] As a kid with a painful disease my learning curve was a bit sharper than most, and like Willie, I learned early that no matter how difficult people make things appear, the truth is simple. So, my "Willieism" for this chapter is one simple truth. Health requires effort every day. There is no free ride. I said the truth is simple, not that it was easy to hear!

The effort involved in healing your life isn't the hamster-on-a-wheel effort we've become so accustomed to in the modern world. I'm talking about pure effort, without wasted energy. "What is hamster-on-a-wheel effort?" you might ask. Look around you; it is like looking for water while swimming in the ocean. We've become so immersed that it's hard to see. Our busy lives are filled with driving here and there, shopping for stuff, taking care of the stuff we acquire, worrying about losing our stuff, working so hard at jobs we don't really like so we can buy more stuff, moving from place to place and from activity to activity. And it keeps starting earlier; these days if you don't have your kids involved in soccer at the age of three, they'll be left behind. Not long ago I counted the number of extra-curricular activities a friend's son was involved in and I stopped counting at seven. So many of my peers are worried that they are getting Alzheimer's disease because they are feeling more forgetful. I remind them that we are not meant to keep track of 37 things at once. "Stop the madness!" I want to yell sometimes. Of course if I did, people would think I was the crazy one. I'm not saying that I haven't fallen prey to this modern epidemic. It has taken me eleven years of hard effort to succeed at being a type B person, and I still sometimes slip. I know I'm slipping when I get up in the morning and feel the need to plan six things before I get out of bed.

Luckily for me pain and joint swelling were a cure for the hamster-on-a-wheel disease, and I've learned what pure effort looks like. When it takes all your might to put a piece of salmon in the toaster oven, you quickly learn where you waste your efforts. It usually comes in the form of things we think we should do, are too ashamed to ask help with, activities that

---

[33] Nelson, W., & Pipkin, T. (2006). The man In the Mirror. In *The Tao of Willie: A guide to the happiness in your heart.* (p. 98) New York: Gotham Books.

leave us exhausted or that we forget the next day. Have you ever asked a friend what they've been up to and they can't remember? There's a sign. How about people who get anxious when they have free time, people who quickly fill up empty space with activity? Effort wasters.

Pure effort has pure intention behind it. It involves being honest with yourself about who you are and what you really want. Once you have this knowledge, as Willie says, the rest is mostly a creative use of adjectives. At one point in my life I had to honestly admit that I was a young woman who was in a serious physical situation. Like it or not, I lived with intense pain and movement was difficult. What I really wanted, besides the obvious, was to continue to serve, to be of use. I knew that for this to happen I had to give my body the rest it desperately needed. During those years I spent a lot of time reading, learning to nap, getting massages, and cooking and eating good food. These activities gave me the energy I needed to write a book for other people with rheumatoid arthritis. Writing this book helped me turn the lemon my life had become into lemonade, helping others with rheumatoid arthritis so life didn't have to be so hard for them.

The pure effort that you put forth changes with the ebb and flow of your life, and you have to be willing to change your habits right along with it. Who you are never changes, but what you do should. Happily, the level of pain I live with has lessened over time, and as it did, I have been able to put more effort into traveling, socializing, and helping others in different ways. The better you get at not wasting effort the easier it is to live the life you want. When you begin to recognize yourself within all the activities you do, you'll know that you've arrived.

"Fall down seven times, get up eight." –Japanese Proverb[34]

This well-known proverb has been quoted many ways and was immortalized in popular culture with a Converse sneaker commercial featuring NBA player Dwayne Wade. The commercial shows Wade making repeated, valiant efforts to score a basket, and falling time and time again. Finally there is a close-up of him belly down on the game floor, with the Look on his face, and he gets up and scores. We all know the Look; we often see it in Hollywood movies. The hero keeps getting beaten

---

[34] Japanese sayings:. (n.d.). Retrieved from http://www.cs.cmu.edu/~fgandon/miscellaneous/japan/

down by the bad guy, and just as we are beginning to wonder if he really is our hero he gives us the Look. Then we know that all is right in the world and sure enough, our hero gets up and starts kicking some bad guy butt. Such a popular Hollywood theme would not be so popular if we all didn't relate to it in some way. It also wouldn't be so popular if we didn't want to believe in it. Real life is rarely as dramatic and as simplistic as the movies but for both this is true; success rarely happens on the first try. The only way to truly know the outcome is by giving up. Give up and you are guaranteed to fail.

I'm fascinated by stories of dramatic remissions from terminal and chronic illnesses. People who succeed at ridding themselves of so-called undefeatable illnesses are anomalies, but not as rare as one might think. Because there is no way to quantify how healing happens, the medical community doesn't invest many resources in investigating further. Outside the medical community, however, there have been attempts at documenting credible spontaneous remissions. The Institute of Noetic Sciences has published 3,500 well-documented cases of them. At the bare minimum 3,500 people have walked away from terminal diseases. This is enough for anyone to stop asking "Why me?" and start asking "Why not me?"

"How long should you try? Until." –Jim Rohn[35]

When I hear of dramatic healings there is one thing that I can't help but think about. Before Jean-Pierre Bely was cured of his multiple sclerosis at the age of 51 in Lourdes, France (a place popular for Catholic Pilgrimage and miraculous healings since the Virgin Mary was said to appear in 1858), how many previous attempts had he made to heal himself? The miracle of his healing may have occurred on September 10, 1987, but I would bet a very large sum of money that he didn't wake up one day and think, "Maybe I'll go to Lourdes and see if I can miraculously heal myself." I can almost guarantee that Mr. Bely had woken up every day for a very long time asking, "What can I do today to help myself to heal?" One day, years into this process, he decided it was time to go to Lourdes. I'm not trying to downplay the miraculous in any way – quite the opposite. What I want to point out is that even miracles take effort. If Mr.

---

[35] 7 Must-Read Life Lessons from Jim Rohn. (n.d.). Retrieved from http://www.mrselfdevelopment.com/2010/02/7-life-lessons-from-jim-rohn

Bely hadn't kept trying, he never would have ended up in Lourdes on the day he was meant to heal. The true hero never gives up.

A few years ago I was at a medical education conference listening to a lecture about chronic pain. That day I learned a lot of great information about what happens physiologically in the body of someone with chronic pain. But I will never forget one slide that came up. It was a picture of a kitchen counter full of supplements. The doctor who was giving the lecture showed this slide as an example of how desperate people in pain become. According to this doctor, these poor people will try anything –even shocking I know, herbs. They will spend hundreds of dollars buying herbs that may or may not help. As I looked at the slide I wanted to sink into my seat. The picture could have been taken in my kitchen. Actually, my counter would have been more full. My chagrin at being one of these desperate people was quickly replaced, however, with pride. In that moment I realized what that counter full of herbs truly represented. It represented strength and hope. It represented someone who was making an effort, despite long odds, to stop their pain. The person who bought all those herbs was not a poor, desperate soul. They were someone on their way to a better life. Back to Willie, who says, "You can't fail every time."

A few months ago I was on a mountain bike ride. I was headed up a hill that seemed endless. I kept telling myself, "Just around the corner and I'll be there," which of course didn't turn out to be the case. At one point I had to walk my bike, and then I skidded over a rock and almost fell. One false summit after another and I began to get frustrated. "Are you kidding me?!" I asked myself as I stubbornly refused to turn around. In the midst of my frustration, I began to laugh. "This is a good metaphor for life," I thought. Nobody ever said it was going to be easy. Of course mountain biking is not as daunting as life because, with the proper maps and background research you will know what you are in for. You can find out just how far you'll have to climb and how many miles you'll have to pedal. There may not be a precise road map to your life, but there is a key. The key is to keep trying and remain unattached to the outcome.

Remain unattached to the outcome. Sounds like a Zen Koan, and believe me, just as hard to grasp. Asking me to be unattached to ridding myself of pain and swelling is like asking my dog Jasper to "just say no" to a deer leg he finds on the trail. However, what I've learned over the years is that with patience it can be done. Remaining unattached to the outcome is something that needs to be experienced instead of talked about, but since this is a book, I'll do my best. Let me begin with a story, maybe my own Zen Koan.

> *One day Kat wakes up and looks at her knees. "Knees!" she says. "You are very troublesome. Why do you pain me so?"*
>
> *Her knees reply, "We are made to move, and today we will." She gets out of bed. Sure enough, her knees move and she begins to walk. She is so mad at her knees that she walks fast just to spite them.*
>
> *The next day Kat wakes up and looks at her knees. "My beautiful knees!" she says. "You are perfect and don't hurt me. What did I do to deserve knees as wonderful as you?"*
>
> *Her knees reply, "We are made to move and today we will." She gets out of bed. Sure enough her knees move and she begins to walk. She is so happy she walks fast and begins to run just to enjoy them.*

The benefit of remaining unattached is that you don't have to be trapped on a runaway rollercoaster ride of emotions. Unattached doesn't mean uncaring. It is the most caring act of all, because it leaves behind your ego. It means that you acknowledge just how big the universe is and how small you are. Small, yet not unimportant. Your efforts may not lead to your destination in the way you think they should, or in the timing you've planned for, but your best efforts always count.

A few months ago I was talking to my friend Staci. We have our best conversations on the phone or in the bathroom when one of us in in the tub; this time I was on the phone with her while in the tub, which meant the conversation was going to be really good. Not that I was attached to that, of course. I was telling her everything that I'd been doing for the past few months on behalf of my healing. "Pippi," she said (yes she calls me Pippi), "With all that you are doing, you are guaranteed to have an impact on your health!" "She's right," I thought, "And I never even gave myself an ultimatum for what had to happen." Keep trying, keep moving, and you are bound to get somewhere. Effort counts.

So, if you aren't attaching to an outcome, what are you supposed to do? This is where intention comes in. Every action has an intention behind it. The intention is the aim that guides the action. If you put on a sweater, your aim is to warm yourself. Buy a birthday gift, and your intention is to show your love for someone. The intention comes first. Having an intention for your life will serve to guide your actions. It will also help keep you actions pure, without wasted effort. Some wise people say that the intention is more important than what you actually do. The feeling around the intention will spur you to action, and that is what counts.

Many spiritual teachers talk about the idea of manifesting what you desire. They call it a variety of things, including the "Law of Attraction," "Intention Manifestation," and "The Law of Detachment." Each teacher has a slightly different approach, but what they all say is that it is necessary to visualize what you want, write it down, imagine it as if it were true, feel it deep inside, believe it will happen, and keep your thoughts aligned with this vision. Have gratitude in the moment, and then tackle the hard part: trust that the manifestation of your desire will be revealed in the right way and time for your highest good.

A fun way to try these ideas out is by creating a vision board. This involves getting a bunch of magazines, a big piece of construction paper, markers, and tape or glue. You then think about what it is you want your life to look like (or an aspect of your life like career or relationship) and you go to town cutting out pictures and words that represent it. After you have filled your vision board, you put it up where you can look at it often and work toward making your dream come true.

My favorite story about a vision board is this one. I have a good friend, Kip, who happens to be an awesome hairstylist. He was the person who discovered that with the right touch and some hair gel I can actually have Shirley Temple curls. We have great conversations as he transforms my hair, and one day I discovered that another amazing talent he has is manifesting. I told him that something on my vision board was about to happen and asked him if he'd ever made one. Kip proceeded to tell me that a few years ago he made a vision board about the person he was going to marry. He had a diamond ring on the board, a picture of the little girl they'd have together, and many more details about his future lover. A year later he realized that he was gay. When Kip realized he was gay, he looked at his vision board and thought, "What a waste of time." Not so fast. A few months later he met Will, who has a daughter, and is everything that Kip put on his board except for the fact that his partner is a he. "I feel like I imagined him into being," said Kip. All I could say was, "Wow!" Last year they were married and Kip wears a diamond ring.

In my own life I've never had such a dramatic result from a vision board, but I have always been happily surprised at what happens in my life whenever I do one. The reason that vision boards work so well for me is that they are fun. I feel like a kid in kindergarten when I'm doing them, which takes away the pressure. Later, looking at the pictures and the words I've created I always feel pleasure. Writing down an affirmation or specific desire, on the other hand, feels like a demand to me. "By September 10, 2013, I will have a flexible job that gives me $100,000 a year and two months vacation." Is it just me or does this have a whiff of "I am Master of the Universe?" I'm sure writing these desires down works well for many people; I just know that the more lighthearted I can feel, the easier it is to be grateful and in the flow of my life. Which leads me back to my last point. It's not what you do that matters as much as how you feel about what you do.

Over the years, I've struggled a lot with the concept of manifestation. I don't agree with some of the ideas I've heard about and I always end up thinking, "If this really worked wouldn't everyone be a perfectly healthy millionaire in a great relationship?" I was once listening to a Wayne Dyer audiobook and he got me so mad I found myself alone in my car yelling at him as he continued to talk. What got me so riled up was his idea that disease has no place in the body. If you are in line with the divine, according to Mr. Dyer, disease will not find its way into your body. He came to this conclusion after telling a story about a friend of his who had undergone a hip replacement and told him, "In a year I know the other hip will have to be replaced. By the way, as a lifelong runner you'll be getting arthritis too and be in my predicament in a few years." Wayne responded that he would never get arthritis. He would just not let that idea into his head and then it would never manifest. "Wow, okay," I thought. "How easy it is for someone who's never had to live with chronic disease to say." I was so mad I would've called him then and there to give him a piece of my mind if I'd had his number.

Wayne Dyer is a very wise person and he has positively influenced the lives of a great many people, including mine. But my take on illness and disease is different than his. My experience with forty-two years of living with pain has shown me that pain has been the greatest teacher I ever could have imagined. It is part of the yin and yang of the universe. It has a very valuable place here on earth, regardless of how uncomfortable it is. To say that disease is not part of the divine plan is like believing you can be a wise monkey by putting your hands over your eyes, ears, and mouth. Yes, it is true that we all want to be happy, healthy, loved, and abundant. But in my experience, unease is the catalyst that brings these things to fruition.

Judging disease will keep you stuck. When your body or life doesn't feel good it is a waste of effort to wish the discomfort away; only by paying attention will you gain the opportunity to learn what is driving the discomfort in the first place. The tendency to judge and suppress discomfort is rife in today's society, especially permeating modern medicine. Dr. Martin Rossman, one of the pioneers in the field of imagery, and one of the few doctors who understands this, uses a wonderful analogy with his patients. He asks them, "If your 'check oil' light went on in your car, would you drive it to the nearest automotive repair shop and have them remove the light?" The obvious answer is, "Of course not, I'd have them check the oil!" He then asks, "Why do you let your doctor do this to your body when you have a physical symptom?" When did we start thinking we could outsmart the walking miracle that is our body? Denying the value of the messages it gives us every day will only serve to keep us right where we are, stridently declaring that we know what's best as we limp down the path of our lives. Eventually the wise choice will emerge. We will embrace the lesson and watch as our life transforms.

"If you think you are too small to make a difference, try sleeping with a mosquito." – Dalai Lama XIV[36]

---

[36] This quote is a paraphrase of the original Dalai Lama quote as discussed in this website. Pappas, J. (2011, July/August). The Top Ten Dalai Lama Quotes...Mistranslated. Retrieved from http://www.elephantjournal.com/2011/07/the-top-ten-dalai-lama-quotes-mistranslated/

Truer words have never been spoken. Every action, decision, and thought in our head has a ripple effect that can extend endlessly without our knowledge. A kind word to a stranger spoken with a smile can change his bad day into a good one. When he gets to his job, perhaps as a loan officer in a bank, he decides to give the young woman coming in without much credit a chance. This young woman goes on to start a business working with disadvantaged kids, using native myths and legends to inspire and encourage them to live with purpose. Every one of those kids moves on in life with an inner confidence and strength that helps them to create healthy relationships and communities. The people they affect then affect others and it goes on- all because you said something nice to a stranger one day. Nice fantasy, right? Try sleeping with a mosquito and then see if you still believe small things can't make a big difference.

You don't often get the opportunity to see where your ripples flow, but when you do it can blow your mind. A few years ago I was working at the Salt Lake City Veterans Hospital. One day I received a referral for a guy who needed replacement compression gloves. That day, instead of following doctors' orders exactly, I used the wiggle room afforded to me as an occupational therapist and did a more thorough evaluation. I did this because my client had idiopathic (meaning a disease of unknown cause) swelling of his hands that wasn't changing despite multiple tests and doctor visits. He also had a litany of other issues including pain, arthritis, fibromyalgia, depression, and nerve damage. When I first met him he talked like an auctioneer – fast, almost manic, seemingly never taking a breath. I got tired just listening to him. I asked him how his sleep was and he replied, "I'm lucky to get five hours." Not surprising, I thought. His body was so ramped up I was happy to hear he got five hours at all.

So instead of handing him a couple of compression gloves and escorting him out the door, I started working with him. Exercises for his hands, electrical therapy point stimulation for his pain and nervous system, relaxation exercises for his mind, and throughout it all we talked. He became a good friend. Over time I could see changes. The miserable guy who was in intense pain, only had a few real friends, and called himself worthless, took mindfulness classes. He began to use his body more, both with exercising and helping others (including myself) with house and car projects. Turns out he is a jack-of-all-trades, has a sharp wit, and a charismatic personality. He is now working with other veterans who are suicidal and/or struggling in other ways. His smart aleck personality isn't the perfect fit for the by-the-book mentality of the Veterans Administration, but he is the most popular mentor they have. He still has over a hundred guns, but no longer contemplates using one on himself. I am extremely proud of him and proud to call him my friend. The lives he is changing will put me to shame, all because one day I decided not to follow doctors' orders to a T.

One of the many gifts of life is the mystery that surrounds it. The greatest minds alive still haven't agreed about some of the most fundamental questions; does consciousness live in the brain; what is time, space, and matter, what is reality, when did advanced civilization begin, who built the pyramids; with each answer we discover ten new questions. This is true for the human body and our individual experience as well. Healing requires stepping into the unknown because it is the known that created ill health. This is what keeps so many people ill for years and lifetimes; they are afraid to take the leap of faith required for health. Instead, if you can hold lightly to your vision allowing for the greater wisdom to emerge within and through you, and remain present with the lessons that your current situation is offering, you can move towards true health. Remember Kip; he allowed the higher understanding of his true nature to be revealed to him and in doing so he found his true love.

The Six Perfections, or paramitas, are guides for those who practice Mahayana Buddhism. They are virtues to be cultivated to bring one to enlightenment. The Six Perfections describe our true nature. They are: Generosity, Ethical Conduct, Patience, Concentration, Wisdom, and Enthusiastic Effort. Enthusiastic Effort is the perfection that enables the attainment of the others. With joyous effort and enthusiastic perseverance, we can see failure as a step toward success, danger as an inspiration for courage, and affliction as another opportunity to practice wisdom and compassion. Sometimes I think that pure effort is the only thing that matters: effort that reflects a humble attitude, has a listening ear, and is in constant communication with the higher wisdom that surrounds us.

MOVEMENT

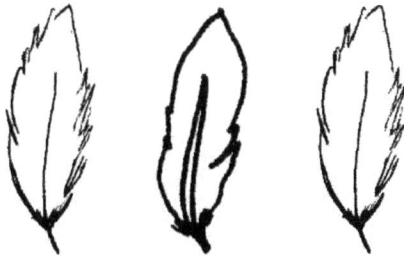

"Life is like riding a bicycle. To keep your balance you must keep moving."

- Albert Einstein[37]

---

[37] Albert Einstein Site Online. (2012, January 8). Retrieved from http://www.alberteinsteinsite.com/quotes/einsteinquotes.html

Movement is no stranger to those of us who live with chronic disease. Unfortunately, this movement often seems like one step forward and three steps back. The insidious specter of the progression of disease never fully escapes the imagination once the possibilities are placed there. The moment-to-moment experience is never boring, but often overwhelming: the movement intentionally created by efforts to reign in the disease; the physical movement required for maintaining strength and quality of life, and the ever-changing thoughts and emotions that reflect the enormity of the task at hand. Movement is no stranger to those of us who live with chronic disease.

Ironically, one of the most challenging aspects to living with a disease, especially a painful one like rheumatoid arthritis, is the difficulty of movement that ensues once the pain takes hold. It's like riding an unbroken horse that is bucking and resisting all over the place and all you can do is freeze and hold on tight. There is chaotic movement swirling inside you; you are in the midst of it wondering what, if anything, is under your control. Within this chaos, how does one create a life that has meaning, one that reflects who you are?

I've struggled with this question for much of my life. It takes an internal core of steel to remember that the broken, crippled body you are carrying around does not reflect your spirit. When the pain makes you so tired you can barely see straight in the middle of a family reunion, it can be hard to remember that the real you is a social butterfly who revels in the company of loved ones. When this body remains gimpy for years on end and life begins to shrink, there is nowhere to move but inside. This is when you finally realize that despite how it may feel as you are perched on your bucking horse, there is movement that you have a choice in. Every minute of every day you are choosing whether to move into fear or hope, faith or despair, gratitude or resentment, pity or empowerment. Ultimately, this is the movement that counts.

"We cannot direct the wind but we can adjust the sails."
–Bertha Calloway[38]

---

[38] This quote has been attributed to Bertha Calloway, Dolly Parton, and Thomas S. Monson among others. A quote by Bertha W. Calloway. (n.d.). Retrieved from http://www.goodreads.com/quotes/377394-we-cannot-direct-the-wind-but-we-can-adjust-our

The movements of nature are evident all around us. They influence each one of us; the waxing and waning of the moon is a beautiful example of this. Scientists may still be debating the lunar effect, but people who work in hospitals or law enforcement have no doubts. When I worked in a locked Alzheimer's care facility I knew exactly when the full moon had arrived. Each month on that day I'd walk into work and be greeted by at least five cute little men and women banging at the door, wanting to go out. Most of them had lost the ability to talk, but not the urge to escape when the moon began to call them.

If we watch nature something becomes clear. Nature moves in cycles; even time isn't linear. So why do humans, obviously part of the natural world, demand a linear existence? If we aren't going somewhere, we are planning our next move. We love to set goals and are taught to break down big goals into smaller ones so that we can chart our progress forward. We teach a linear version of evolution to our children even though science long ago debunked this idea. The 2012 calendar year "End of the World" phenomenon misunderstood the date as potentially marking the end of time, when it really was marking the end of a cycle in the Mesoamerican long-count calendar. Our stubborn refusal to acknowledge the cyclical nature of existence will always end in a lament when things don't move forward in the way we want them to.

The particular disease that has been a part of me for most of my life is so starkly cyclical it can be comical. I can literally feel the swelling begin to creep into my joints until I begin to wonder if I could stick a pin in them and pop them like a balloon. In a matter of hours the movement of this invisible disease can alter my life, and prevent me from moving. My best-laid plans will have to be changed and my small ninety-five pound body becomes a ginormous load to carry around. Every movement I make becomes hesitant and is accompanied by a gritting of the teeth. Then, just as I begin to wonder how much more pain I can take, it begins to lift. My invisible enemy that is called rheumatoid arthritis begins to retreat and I am granted a much needed reprieve.

For many years I fought this fact of my life with all my strength. Like most people who believe that movement should always be forward, I would feel personally thwarted every time the tugging at my joints began, and I would judge each new development harshly. "Damn arthritis," I would rage at myself. When I wasn't angry, I would be wondering what I did wrong to create the latest round of swelling. Over and over I would be held captive to the whims of my irascible disease. For years I held a vision of being trapped in a whirlpool, treading water so I wouldn't drown, but going nowhere. This vision haunted me on days that the arthritis was particularly active. I felt trapped by this disease that was preventing me from living my life, from moving forward in the way I wanted, and constantly impeding all my careful plans. The more I struggled to move forward, the more frustrating and depressing life became. Over time, I finally began to understand something. The real enemy was never the rheumatoid arthritis; it was my toxic reaction to it. I finally began to, as Bono famously sings, "play Jesus to the lepers in my head."

"Developing inner values is much like physical exercise. The more we train our abilities, the stronger they become. The difference is that, unlike the body, when it comes to training the mind, there is no limit to how far we can go." -Dalai Lama[39]

Unraveling the misguided notions I had been carrying around for so many years was a process, one that continues today. Each step I take in this process frees my mind, which ultimately is the most important freedom there is. Living with grace, especially when times are tough, is true wisdom. The Dalai Lama speaks about the limitations of our body, and the unlimited nature of the spirit and mind; this notion has transformed my life. Movement is always happening, and we can use the movements outside of ourselves as fuel to create a greater wisdom inside. As I've said many times the truth is simple and the truth is; life is meant to be enjoyed, not resisted. You can decide to enjoy your life even in the midst of great challenge and discomfort, Letting go of resistance will take you there.

"Reject your sense of injury and the injury itself disappears. "
-Marcus Aurelius[40]

[39] Lama, D. (2011, December 30). Developing inner values is much like physical exercise. The more we train our... Retrieved from https://plus.google.com/+DalaiLama/posts/gXfBNq9WBaA
[40] Reject your sense of injury and the injury itself disappears. (2011, November 30). Retrieved from http://philosiblog.com/2011/11/30/reject-your-sense-of-injury-and-the-injury-itself-disappears/

I once heard someone say, "You can only lean one way at once." It hit home because at the time I was leaning into self-pity. My life had once again become a bad country song, and honestly, I was growing weary. When I heard those words I thought to myself, "So how is the self-pity going for you? Liking it yet?" Then I felt ashamed. I had to admit feeling ashamed didn't work much better, so I laughed. Only then did I back off and decide to make the nourishing choice for myself. I took a good hard look at the events that had transpired. I admitted that most of them weren't my fault; they fell under the category of, "Life Happens." Other things were the result of choices I had made, misguided maybe, but the best I could do at the time. Where I had gone wrong was in my reactions. As soon as life began to move into stormy sailing I felt my trust, faith, and hope fade. I no longer believed I was being taken care of and began to tell myself that God had forgotten about me. This, unfortunately, is one of the sad and yes, pathetic stories I've told myself over the years. When my pain has gotten the best of me I've tended to think, "Where is that magical healing force and why is it passing me by?" Then I find myself leaning into victimhood. My poor, pitiful circumstance takes over my mind, and my psyche. This happens until I get tired of feeling this way and decide to lean in the other direction.

Gary Zukov puts it this way: you have the choice between love and fear; choose love. The more I take his sage advice, the better I feel. I'm not saying this is easy. In some circumstances it can be really hard, but the following is a story that can inspire one to do it.

There was a beautiful woman who loved to ride horses. She rode every day feeling the wind through her hair, hearing her horse's nostrils flaring as he got excited, smelling the fresh sage. One day her new horse was startled by a rabbit and bucked her off. She broke her neck and became paralyzed. As she lay in bed recovering, she found herself wanting to die. All day, hopelessness consumed her as she thought of how her life had changed and all she had lost, until one day she woke up and decided to change. From that day forward she gave herself thirty minutes to grieve and then she stopped. She began to assess her situation. She moved into her new reality and began to plan her life as a quadriplegic. As her mind shifted, so did her life. Yours will too, the more often you choose to lean the other way.

You can lean the other way in every situation you find yourself in. When you are talking with a friend and find yourself gossiping, you can stop and lean back into right speech. When you get irritated at your mother for hen-pecking your life, you can decide to appreciate the fact that you have a loving mother who cares. When you find yourself thinking how unlucky you are, you can choose to remember all the amazing things that have happened to you during your life. When you are feeling like you are the only unlovable person left on the planet, you can begin to count just how many people really do love you, and yes you can count your dog. You can only lean one way at once. Choose wisely.

"The least movement is of importance to all nature. The entire ocean is affected by a pebble." –Blaise Pascal[41]

Small shifts make a huge difference. The moment I decided to stop trying to figure out the cause of every change in my body, I freed up an immense amount of emotional energy that I could use to foster gratitude and joy in my life. Keeping my thoughts on the present situation instead of comparing each event to the past or worrying about the future enables me to take advantage of each moment. You never get the moments of your life back. Each one is unique, so why waste these precious moments fretting? There is so much to be gained from moving with the tides of life, and for cherishing each moment as if it were your last, because it really is the last time you will have that particular one.

When we are always trying to move away from pain and towards pleasure we miss the point; it all has value. I don't actually believe the notion that life will keep presenting us with the same lesson until we learn it. Instead I think that once we learn it we don't see it as a lesson anymore. It ceases to trigger us in the way it used to, and we are free. My joints haven't stopped swelling now that I don't rage against them, but as they swell I recognize that it is time for me to move into a more internal enjoyment of life instead of expending a lot of physical energy that I really don't have.

A few months ago I moved to Bayfield, Colorado, near Durango. Newly single, I decided to do what most twenty-first century

---

[41] Blaise Pascal quote. (n.d.). Retrieved from
http://www.brainyquote.com/quotes/quotes/b/blaisepasc159856.html

single people do: go on match.com. Whenever you do this you have to have a sense of humor because, in case you haven't discovered this yet, people are strange. I quickly learned why people from Durango are nicknamed "Durangotangs." They are beyond fit. The first guy had to do an hour and a half run before we met for a two-hour hike. The next one was up at six a.m. the morning of our date so he could get an intense yoga workout in. He then proceeded to hike me up a mountain. Halfway through he informed me that he was timing us and we were way behind schedule. When we were driving back I innocently asked him what possessed him to take me for a grueling hike on a first date. His offhand reply was, "You seemed like the hiking type, and besides, this is the easiest hike I do." I must qualify this description by adding that they were both perfectly nice men, and I'm sure there is a great "Durangotangette" out there waiting patiently for them. Of course she's probably climbing a mountain right now while she's waiting. The point of this story isn't to make fun of the intense nature of Durango singles, (okay, not completely) but to remind you that sometimes epiphanies come during the most unlikely of situations.

While I was hiking up the mountain with Sam he began talking about his mountain climbing adventures. Apparently he had lived in Washington State and had once hiked up a mountain with Ed Visteurs, an amazing high-altitude mountaineer and the first American to climb all fourteen of the world's highest peaks without oxygen. If I hadn't already realized this, it became clear that Sam was no slouch in the fitness department after he told me about knowing Ed. Just for kicks, Sam and his buddies used to run up mountain peaks in Washington, come down and do it all over again. As he was telling me about his many extreme adventures, he said something that could have come out of the mouth of a yogi (maybe all the yoga was working): "I can go on an eight-hour hike and climb four thousand feet of elevation. Maybe I'll pass an overweight guy slowly walking one quarter of the distance and really, in the end we will be doing the same amount of work." Sam, who only stopped to take in the view when I insisted, had somehow noticed something that 98% of the people who are similarly physically blessed never will. It's not how far you can go that matters, it's the effort you put into your movement. Spending time comparing yourself to those around you will only serve to crush or feed your ego.

You can ask many people with chronic disease and they will tell you the same thing: it is easy to take the ability to move for granted until you no longer can. When you are physically blessed, often you will personalize this blessing to the point where you forget that your effortless physicality was given to you, not earned. There is a thoughtlessness that comes with this, and a disconnection. This separateness is starkly felt by those of us who can't take our bodies' efforts for granted anymore. Our movements may look less heroic, but the effort involved is often more so.

I think one reason why so many people who have physical challenges opt out of participating in exercise completely is that they have a hard time accepting their new reality. A whopping 70% of people with arthritis don't exercise. Of course, there is the fact that when you have arthritis exercise hurts, which is a huge disincentive, but I've also heard people say that because they can't do the activities they used to enjoy they gave up trying anything. This is one of the most disheartening things I hear from my patients, because it is a sign of resignation. Our bodies are made to move, and denying this innate urge is an invitation to a slow death. I think I'm lucky because I'm someone who actually really likes to exercise, and I'm also not a competitive sort. Sure, I don't like to be left behind, and I definitely don't like to be left out, but being the fastest or strongest isn't my life's goal. Instead, I enjoy moving my body every day, at whatever pace it needs.

In our goal-oriented society there is a strong drive to always move towards improvement – bigger, better, stronger is always more desirable. If you can do 10,000 steps a day, then, why, you'd better do 12,000. If you have a cellphone, then why aren't you getting a smartphone? If you like drinking a twenty-ounce Slurpee, then of course you'll like a thirty-two ounce Slurpee even more. This obsession has had significant negative consequences. The humungous Slurpee makes you humungous, needing the latest gadget makes you a slave to always needing to work so you can afford it, and yes, there is such a thing as too much exercise. Over exercising has many deleterious effects on the body, including insomnia, heart failure, a weakened immune system, and a loss of lean muscle mass. Most amateur athletes are so oblivious to this reality that they constantly injure themselves, and they joke about taking daily doses of Vitamin I (Ibuprofen). This obsession is the shadow of the drive towards innovation, the creative process of improving technology, or coming up with ideas to improve life for individuals and society. We've forgotten that sometimes its okay to move for movement's sake, even when it won't result in bragging rights. It's easy to see why many people with chronic physical conditions choose to opt out entirely from exercise instead of joining this manic race.

When it comes to handling the pressure towards incessant "improvement," like the Dalai Lama I've chosen the middle way. Sometimes it can be hard to explain to people why I can't do a long bike ride with them when I just went out a week before and climbed a mountain. There is a learning curve for people who don't live with chronic disease for understanding those who do, and when you are the teacher, sometimes you need a day off. So, on my bad pain days my companion will more often than not be my little right-hand man Jasper, who is my goofy gentle giant of a dog. He never asks me to explain, doesn't give me pitying looks, or tell me to take pain medication. I don't have to spend time allaying his concerns about how bad my limp is, or have a discussion about what I am going to do to make it better. I don't have to bite my lip when I really just want to say, "If I knew the answers I'd be a billionaire and living on my own island instead of talking to you about your endless questions!" He just stays with me, grinning because we are together. While I watch Jasper follow his nose and try not to get dizzy, I'm glad I can limp or walk slowly in solitude. I truly enjoy these experiences, even though from the outside looking in they are not ideal, because there is no pressure to perform or to take care of other people's concerns. Maybe I'm failing to travel faster, longer, and harder with each passing day, but I'm also not allowing any day to pass by un-enjoyed.

Movement for movement's sake is win-win. You are serving your body's need to move, and you are staying present in your mind instead of comparing your movement to yesterday or tomorrow. One thing I love about going to Bikram Yoga is hearing the instructor say, "Do your yoga using the body you came with today. Don't compare yourself with your neighbor or with what you accomplished last time you were here." Every time I hear these words, I relax.

"The human mind is like a drunken monkey ... that's been stung by a bee ..." -Bikram Choudhury[42]

---

[42] Love.Life.Yoga. (2014, July/August). Retrieved from https://bikramyogamusings.wordpress.com/tag/om-chant/

I love the term "Monkey Mind." It is used by meditation teachers to describe the constant chatter that people hear when they first attempt to clear their mind. Anyone who has ever attempted meditation will relate to the experience of closing your eyes, taking a few deep breaths, and hearing a three-ring circus in your head. Do this a few times and you'll begin to wonder who's in charge: your looney mental chatter, or your higher wisdom. For most of us, looney prevails. The practice of sitting and simply listening to your incessant chatter is a practice in itself, because you'll quickly realize which thoughts are in control. For me it's worry, usually unrealistic, or fantasy, sadly, again usually unrealistic. Once you begin to observe your thoughts, you will notice how they make you feel. Often when I do this I feel my thoughts in my heart or gut. Now you're closer to moving into a deeper understanding of yourself, how your mind and body changes along with the thoughts in your head. People are very aware of the changes in their outer world, but their inner world is a vast, unexplored territory until they begin to visit regularly.

A while ago, as I began my own inner quest, I began to notice the mental habits of others along with my own. What I observed made me laugh because I realized why women get such a bad rap for being emotional. Around that time it seemed as if all my girlfriends were having man trouble. One after the other, they obsessed to me over the infatuation they felt, the misery of not getting a phone call, what he meant when he said he had a lot on his plate, or the euphoria that resulted when he told her how amazing she was. As I observed them, I realized that the problem wasn't that they were overemotional. It was how seriously they took the emotions they felt. They were caught up in the emotional drama that their feelings caused and they were creating more drama by holding onto those feelings instead of releasing them and moving on to the next moment. They failed to recognize their emotions as important information, but not the whole story.

From my perspective, the cause of all of this turmoil was not knowing the outcome. So desperate to move into relationship with someone, and so anxious to know if he was "the one," each of my friends forgot one point: being with someone should be fun. And the mystery, if you let it, is part of the fun. Our thoughts and emotions are always in motion, and this motion is what makes up the experience of your life, not the certainty of an end result. I admit that I often peruse the last page of books that I'm reading, but I doubt I'd want to read the last page of my life because I still want to think that has yet to be written. If you can resist the temptation to need proof of outcome for the events in your life you can begin to relax and enjoy it. And even when it's so uncomfortable you can't do this, at least you can sit back, shake your head, laugh, cry, or all three, while you wait for things to change. As my friend Willie Nelson says, "Life is not about how fast you run or how high you climb, but how well you bounce."

Over time it becomes easier to honor the movements and cycles of your body/mind without putting demands on it. This is when you make different choices, and you'll find that these new choices will begin to create a new shape to your life. Sometimes the new shape will be obvious from the outside, and sometimes the difference will be subtle to others but inside you'll feel like a new person. One of the largest shifts I've experienced is how I handle the ups and downs of the cycles of my pain and swelling. I'm almost embarrassed to admit that it took me this long to stop kicking myself when I was down, but, yes, for the majority of my life this is what happened on a regular basis:

I'd begin to wake up in pain every day, usually too early because my body wasn't relaxed, and as I began to move through the day the pain would lessen. I'd continue to go about my daily activities, maybe moving a bit slower, but happy that nobody but me noticed. After a few weeks of this, one day I'd wake up either really sad or having had a particularly bad nightmare. As the day wore on I'd want to cry and eventually something would trigger me and the tears would start. I'd retreat somewhere I knew no one would have to witness this unbecoming scene. As I cried I would feel a jumble of emotions: part relief at not having to hold my tears in anymore, part anxiety about what was going on, part anger at my fate, part fear about what the future held, and part frustration that here I was again. I'd worry about plans that I'd made, imagining myself not getting enough rest or not being able to do the things I told my friends or family I'd be joining them on. Then I'd get resentful, angrier, more frustrated, and extremely worried. I'd rage against my fate, tell myself that I was better off alone because it was easier that way and second guess everything I'd done recently to have possibly caused this situation to occur. I'd keep doing this until my joints decided to give me a break or until I went to the doctor and got a strong medication to help my symptoms. As soon as I felt better, all would be forgotten until the next time, when, like the movie Groundhog Day, it would happen all over again. Never once did I recognize that I was pouring salt into my wounds.

By resisting what was happening to me with my thoughts, and by ignoring what my body needed with my actions, I kept myself stuck. Tenaciously moving in my inflexible pattern of life as I knew it, I was acting out my own nightmare; I was treading water in a whirlpool of my own making. After a lifetime of this I'd finally had enough. I decided that the only way I would ever become healthy in my body was to become flexible in my mind and actions. I had to make different choices if I wanted a different outcome. As Einstein famously said, "The definition of insanity is doing the same thing and expecting a different result."

As usual, once I decide something, there is no going back. As I'm not someone who does things halfway, I moved out of my comfort zone with gusto. I turned all my normal reactions to the situations I found myself in on their head. If I found myself worrying, I told myself, "Everything works out, it will be okay," and I decided to believe this. When my mind turned toward fear, I asked myself, "What is the worst thing that could happen?" When the answer was the scary idea that maybe I'd become a crippled invalid, I thought about what that would actually look like. Could I enjoy my life if this were the case? Would I still be okay? I kept finding that the answer was yes. Instead of letting my emotional reactions to the pain take over and paralyze me, I used them as catalysts for action. I found that I could move into each feeling with genuine curiosity and see clearly how each was helping or hurting me. By not taking my emotions too seriously, they didn't snowball. Instead, they retreated as I moved back into comfort. I've learned to honor the pain and the pleasure, the fear and the relief; neither is better or worse and it's a trap to struggle against them. If I ask my anger, "Hey, what's going on?" it will tell me, and then the conversation is over and I can move on. This invisible movement is the kind that changes lives.

Moving into true health is a process. It takes dogged determination and perseverance. It requires stepping into the unknown. Over and over one needs to take leaps of faith. Sometimes things have to cycle back into extreme discomfort in order to have true insights and deeper understandings. You will be required to move at your own pace, regardless of what is happening outside of you or what is expected from those around you. As you begin to relax into the process, you will perceive the movements of your inner and outer worlds differently, and you will be gently guided to live differently. The safe path will show itself to actually be the dangerous one; the scary path will begin to look more inviting. And you will find yourself at home within the rhythms of your life.

RESILIENCE

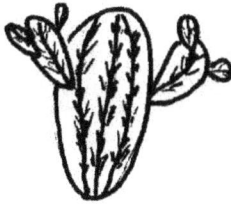

"Look well into thyself; there is a source of strength which will always spring up if thou wilt always look."

–Marcus Aurelius, Meditations[43]

---

[43] Marcus Aurelius. (n.d.). Retrieved from http://izquotes.com/quote/280949

Resilience is the ultimate life skill. Without it a person easily becomes overwhelmed by the many challenges that life dishes out. With it, no challenge is too large. It is also a requirement for living well with chronic disease, which will present challenges on a daily basis. Official definitions of resilience include:

- The act of rebounding or springing back after being stretched or pressed, or recovering strength, spirit, and good humor.
- Experiencing life's challenges and adversities and then not only recovering but improving self-esteem, confidence, happiness, and life skills.
- Unpredicted or markedly successful adaptations to negative life events, trauma, and other forms of risk.

Personally, I like the second definition best as it most closely mirrors my own ideas about resilience. I believe that moving through adversity resiliently will lead to the ability to do it better the next time, and the capacity to be a happier, wiser, and more peaceful person. Being resilient isn't always easy to do, but it is always better than the alternative, which is something to keep in mind on the days when you want to pull the covers back over your head and stay in bed rather than face the day. Resilience is both the most natural habit you can foster in your life and also one that takes much internal fortitude as you resist the contagion of apathy and fear that can so easily find its way to you.

Someone who is searching for inspiration about resilience needs only to walk into nature and open his eyes. Examples of resilience are everywhere: flowers that bloom atop a cactus that gets only two inches of rain every year, a tree that gets split in half by a lightning strike and manages to grow two trunks. The movie March of the Penguins documents a remarkable example of resilience. Emperor penguins travel seventy miles to the only breeding ground in the area where the ice doesn't melt year round. They find a mate, and the female lays one egg. She then carefully transfers it to her partner, who will sit with it for two months as she travels the seventy miles back to the ocean to feed. By this time she has lost half her weight. Once she is strong enough, she travels back to feed her baby while her partner goes back to the ocean. The next year they all turn around to do it again. If you open your eyes and pay attention, you will see that resiliency abounds.

'I saw the angel in the marble and carved until I set him free."
–Michelangelo[44]

The first key to resilience is imagination. What does imagination have to do with resilience? Read the following definitions and then ask that question again.

- The act or power of forming a mental image of something not present to the senses or never before wholly perceived in reality
- Creative ability
- Ability to confront and deal with a problem: resourcefulness
- The thinking or active mind
- A creation of the mind, especially an idealized or poetic creation

You went for a day hike in the mountains. You brought some water, a Cliff bar, and a light jacket. "I'll hike just a bit more," you tell yourself, and when you turn around it is a bit later than you'd anticipated. Suddenly you see a fork in the trail. "I don't remember this," you tell yourself. "Which way did I come up?" Before you know it you are hopelessly lost and it's getting dark. First question- what age group do you want to be: six or under, seven to fifteen, sixteen to thirty, thirty to fifty, or above fifty? Believe it or not, the age group with the highest survival rate in a situation similar to the one I just described is the six or under category. Why, you ask? Because kids haven't forgotten how to be resilient. They don't overthink or stubbornly refuse to believe they've been this careless. When they get cold, they find shelter, when hungry they scavenge for food, and they don't waste their precious energy walking in circles. Most importantly, children haven't lost their ability to imagine their way out of a problem; they don't think of imagination as a silly waste of time, instead they take their imagination seriously.

Can you remember how you used your imagination as a child? I spent time writing stories, watching and drawing animals, and inventing things. Believe it or not, this was great training for a career in occupational therapy. And my ability to call upon my

44 Michelangelo quote. (n.d.). Retrieved from
http://www.brainyquote.com/quotes/quotes/m/michelange161309.htm

imagination as an adult has enabled me to survive big and little challenges, including being lost in the woods.

Here's a story for you:

I had decided to do an overnight camp trip with my friend Staci. We drove two hours east from Salt Lake City into the Uinta Mountains, and as we were unpacking I realized I had forgotten the tent. Luckily, we had her two dogs with us, and Big Dog was both a great heating pad and mellow enough to have no problem with volunteering for the job. That problem solved, Staci and I went for a hike. Close to dark we got lost – so lost that there was nothing to do but have a seat under a tree and consider our options. I decided not to panic; it wasn't cold enough to be worried about frostbite. Instead I looked around, and as I did I watched Staci's other dog Doug. Doug seemed to know where to go. She kept looking at us as she came over to where we were sitting and then trotting away in the same direction. "Staci," I said, "Doug is showing us the way back!" Sure enough, she did. We got back to our campsite in just enough time to snuggle into our sleeping bags next to Big Dog and Doug.

"Life can deal you an amazing hand. Do you play it steady, bluff like crazy or go all in?" –Joe Simpson[45]

Perseverance. When I think of this word I think of the book *Touching the Void*. It is a true story of Joe Simpson, a young climber who broke his leg on the way down from a first ascent of Suila Grande, a treacherous mountain in Peru. Through a series of fortunate and misfortunate events he proceeded to save his own life. He was climbing alpine style, which means he and his partner Simon brought minimal gear and were fully self-supported; no one was waiting at the bottom of the mountain with a radio ready to rescue them if they got into trouble. In fact, except for a casual day hiker they had met on the way to the mountain there was nobody around for miles. So when Joe broke his upper leg and smashed his knee while at 19,000 feet, a small part of him had to be thinking that he was dead. His partner Simon bravely decided to lower him down the mountain with a rope, which meant that he had to dig a seat in the snow and risk being pulled off the mountain himself or suffer severe frostbite as the night fell. All seemed to be going

---

[45] Simpson, J. (2004). *Touching the void* (p. 215). New York: Perennial.

reasonably well with this plan until a storm blew in and visibility fell to nothing. As Simon lowered Joe, all of a sudden the rope got very heavy. Unknowingly he had lowered Joe over a ledge, and Joe was hanging over a huge crevasse, unable to climb up to safety. After many agonizing minutes where Simon felt himself being pulled off the mountain, he did the only thing he could do. He cut the rope.

Joe fell into a huge crevasse and landed on a small ledge, remarkably unhurt except for his original injury, with nowhere to go and nothing to see except for the enveloping darkness that surrounded him. He had a rope, and realized that his choices were to stay there until he died of thirst, or use the rope and lower himself further into the crevasse to see if he could hit bottom. He chose the latter, and began the long rappel down into the unknown. The idea of lowering oneself into a dark hole with no hope of rescue makes my skin crawl, but Joe was able to imagine a possible way out. Sure enough, he ended up at the bottom and was able to see sunlight in the distance. He managed to climb his way out into the sunlight through sheer force of will with two hands and one leg. Once out of the crevasse, Joe still had miles of hiking to do to get back to camp, unsure if anyone would be waiting for him. Because of his broken leg, he literally crawled for miles, hallucinating, in and out of lucidity, but still refusing to give in to his fate. Joe never stopped thinking of solutions to every problem he confronted as he made his way down the mountain. Even at the bleakest moments, when he logically knew that his chances for survival were less than slim, he continued to persevere, to move forward, and this saved his life.

What can we all learn from this? When all else fails, suspend logic and remember to keep trying. There will always be people, scientific evidence, statistics, opinions and schools of thought that weigh against your ability to bounce back from any challenge, but the power of perseverance can defeat them all.

"I haven't failed. I've identified 10,000 ways this doesn't work."
–Thomas Edison[46]

Resilient people have a unique perspective. They believe in their ability to succeed and won't be dissuaded by anyone or

---

[46] Thomas A. Edison quote. (n.d.). Retrieved from
http://www.brainyquote.com/quotes/quotes/t/thomasaed132683.html

anything. The first thing you must do in order to live a resilient life is to believe in yourself. Believe in your ability to face any challenge that comes your way and believe in your capacity to imagine your way through it. The people who survive and learn to thrive in difficult circumstances have dogged determination and the ability to see failure as another step on the ladder of success. Consider this quote from Michael Jordan:

> I have missed more than 9,000 shots in my career. I have lost almost 300 games. On 26 occasions I have been entrusted to take the game winning shot... and I missed. I have failed over and over and over again in my life. And that's precisely why I succeed.[47]

People like Michael Jordan don't see failure as an end, just an excuse to do it right the next time. In the game of basketball or the game of life, there will be many, many, many chances to stand up again after falling, and people who choose to be resilient will be the first to be grateful for another chance.

Over the years I've read many stories of extreme survival written by people who were caught in the middle of war, political strife, or held prisoner and tortured just because they were in the wrong place at the wrong time. They were people who'd been treated so badly by others that you'd expect them to want nothing more than the death and destruction of their captors. Instead they found their way to forgiveness. Their physical scars may have lasted, but their psychological and spiritual wounds were healed through forgiving their enemies. By choosing not to continue the cycle of persecution and hatred, they were able to transmute their suffering into love and compassion, and in doing so they became teachers for all of us.

One heart-wrenching example of this is the genocide in Rwanda in the early 1990's. The two main ethnic groups in Rwanda, the Tutsis and the Hutus, lived in peace until 1923 when Belgian colonists created a ruling class of Tutsis. Animosity began to soar between the groups, and came to a head in 1994 when Hutus gained majority rule and ordered people to kill the Tutsi "cockroaches." Hutus armed themselves with machetes and aimed to kill 1,000 people every 20 minutes. The murder lasted 100 days, during which time 75% of all Tutsis were killed.

47 Michael Jordan quote. (n.d.). Retrieved from
http://www.brainyquote.com/quotes/quotes/m/michaeljor127660.html

Nearly a million people died, over 500,000 women were raped, and over 300,000 children were orphaned. After the bloodbath, the country lay in ruins.

The question of what to do with the perpetrators of the killing loomed large, since it was estimated that it would take 110 years to take everyone to trial. It was decided that Rwanda would go back to its traditional roots, and in 2001 a community justice system called the Gacaca court began. The Gacaca court is designed to promote healing and reconciliation by bringing in the victims and members of the community to speak in front of the perpetrator. The perpetrator then explains himself directly to the families of the victims. Other programs sprung up, including a program where Hutus and Tutsis built houses together for victims of the genocide. Slowly, forgiveness began to blossom throughout Rwanda. People whose entire families were killed were visiting the men who killed them in prison. If you were in Rwanda during this time, you'd see men hugging the murderer of their brother, women sitting down to a meal with the killer of their children, people dancing together, and Hutus and Tutsis marrying. In the space of less than ten years this country torn apart by hatred was transformed by the alchemy of love and forgiveness.

Along with forgiveness, this story reminds us that resilience doesn't happen in a vacuum. We need each other to heal and to be healed. A resilient person doesn't isolate themselves from others for very long. He recognizes that challenging times and trauma should bring us together, not tear us apart, and he finds ways to reach out to others whenever and however he can. Surrounding yourself with friends, family, and those who make you feel good is imperative in living a resilient life. Feeling supported and connected helps one to be more optimistic about life in general, and one's challenges in particular. Sometimes you don't even have to talk about it; all you have to do is bask in the camaraderie and comfort of those who love and care for you, and you begin to feel better.

Optimism is a requirement for a resilient life. Not the rose-colored glasses form of optimism which is just denial in disguise, but the kind that comes from a conscious choice. Abe Lincoln once said, "Most people are about as happy as they make their minds up to be," and he was entirely right. Every situation has many possible outcomes, and until you know for certain that the outcome will be bad, there is no reason to believe this. The ability to re-frame your ideas about your situation is the heart of resiliency. Thinking back to Joe Simpson's story of survival, I know that if at any point during his ordeal he had decided his situation was hopeless, that's what it would have become. Whenever I find myself feeling discouraged, I tell myself that attitude is everything, because in most situations it really is, and I immediately find my attitude becoming more positive. Then I tell myself something the Dalai Lama says. "Choose to be optimistic. It feels better."

The book *Deep Survival, Who Lives, Who Dies, and Why*, by Lawrence Gonzales, describes many stories about people who have and have not survived plane crashes, mountain climbing accidents, and other severe challenges in the outdoors. It also contains much advice for people interested in cultivating their resilience.

Let me expand on a few points he mentions in his writing. How many times have you gotten through a difficult time, sat back on your laurels telling yourself, "Damn I'm good!" only to have life quickly hand you something else to deal with? This has happened to me more times than I care to remember, especially with my ever-changing swollen joints. Celebrating the summit too wholeheartedly is a sure-fire way to find out what a false summit is. It doesn't get easier to bounce back from a flare-up time and time again; in fact, it can get harder. Hope begins to drain out of your body, and the temptation to give in to the thought that you'll never feel better again gets stronger. The question becomes, how do you stay resilient when your body feels so broken, so unyielding? What's a resilient person to do?

The first thing is to stop asking why. It is natural to try to figure out what caused your body to take two steps back, but it's rarely useful. The only time you want to do this is if you are trying a new health or medical regimen, or are tracking symptoms along with other things like exercise, sleep, emotions, or stress. Otherwise the question "Why?" quickly turns into "Why me?" Instead, learn to make the most of any situation, to access inner peace and the knowledge that this, too, shall pass. This is easier said than done, but not impossible. Resiliency is an inside job, and has to stem from a strong inner foundation. If you are in touch with your inner values, a deep understanding of what is most important to you, you will be less likely to be thrown by the curveballs of life. You will be better at keeping harmful emotions in check and staying in alignment with the truth of who you are. You will stay on the right path instead of letting fear drive you to make decisions that you will later regret.

With this in mind, think of how good it feels to acknowledge success with the small steps you are taking to live well. Every so often stepping back and reflecting on helpful actions or behaviors that you've incorporated into your life will build your internal power and resolve. Life is full of false summits, and never giving up is the only path to success.

Using a mantra makes sense when you hear some of the stories survival expert and author Lawrence Gonzales tells. Yossi Ghinsberg, lost while hiking in the Bolivian jungle for three weeks, kept repeating, "Man of action." Steve Callahan, adrift at sea for 76 days, said the word "Survive." For Jerry Long, paralyzed from the neck down after a diving accident, reminding himself daily that "I broke my neck, my neck didn't break me" helps to keep him living with purpose. Mr. Gonzales has his own- "Trust the process." He says, "Once I've gone through the steps of creating a strategy, I continue telling myself to trust that the process will get me where I'm going."[48]

I've had my own over the years. As a young adult I used the slightly masochistic Nike mantra of, "No pain no gain." Although I've moved beyond this belief, at the time it served a very useful purpose, reminding me that pain didn't have to prevent me from moving forward and reaching my goals. Now I have a few other mantras: "The only way to fail is to stop trying," "I am love, I am loved," and "Hurt or heal?" Using a mantra can change your perspective and emotional state immediately, and aid your ability to never give up.

One way that I've been able to ward off despair is my ability to laugh at myself, especially when my situation has reached the level of the absurd and I find myself saying, "You've GOT to be kidding me!" Doctors are famous for gallows humor, a coping technique allowing them to get through a day filled with pain, misfortune and death. The veterans I've worked with who are faring well in their lives, post deployment, are always the ones who have kept their sense of humor. My veteran friend Buck gives this advice: "Breathe deep, Say ahhhhhh, breathe deep, say sh....t, repeat until stress abates." Yes, he is a sailor!

---

[48] Gonzales, Laurence. "Adventure Travel - National Geographic Adventure Magazine." Adventure Travel - National Geographic Adventure Magazine. National Geographic, Aug. 2008. Web. 28 May 2015.

Someone who knows this is J.R. Martinez, a young man who was serving in Iraq in 2003 as an infantryman when the Humvee he was driving hit an improvised explosive device, or IED. He suffered severe smoke inhalation and burns on over 34% of his body. He spent the next 34 months in recovery and underwent 33 surgeries. If anyone had an excuse to stop smiling, he did, but J.R. was raised by a single Mom who always found ways to smile. Through her example he found ways to stay positive and persevere, even when the pain was intense and he didn't want to look in the mirror. J.R. transitioned from a twenty-year-old man who faced a life with the stigma that facial burns can bring and an uncertain future to a successful guy who landed a role on a soap opera – fitting right into the land of the beautiful people – and won a competition in the television show "Dancing with the Stars," which is extremely physically taxing. Then he wrote a best-selling book, and now he's the father of a baby girl. He didn't do this by dwelling on his disfigurement or pain. J.R's success only happened because he never gave up, lost hope, or stopped believing in himself, and he definitely never stopped smiling.

When all else fails, you've got to laugh. Laughter is the best weapon for despair and the best friend of resilience. In my quest to be as resilient as I possibly can, I've found that any excuse to laugh is a good one. And a belly laugh is better than a giggle, but a giggle doesn't hurt. A good cry may be a necessity from time to time, but as far as I'm concerned a smile and a laugh trump a good cry every time.

Be cool. This is another essential tip. Mr. Gonzales says, "Stress changes the shape and chemistry of the brain, resulting in trouble remembering, difficulty completing tasks, and altered behavior. In effect, losing your cool makes you stupid."[49] Anyone who learns to scuba dive is taught two golden rules: (1) always breathe, and (2) never panic. I've seen someone panic under the water and shoot to the surface, risking the bends. I've seen another grab his partner's regulator from her mouth, and yet another start flapping wildly to move away from an eel, kicking and killing the coral reef and wasting precious air. Over the years I've had my share of outdoor adventure, and whenever I embark on a fun, yet potentially dangerous activity I'm always taking note of the people I'm with. Who will I be able to count on when things don't go according to plan (because

---

[49] Gonzales, L. (2008, August). Adventure Travel - National Geographic Adventure Magazine. Retrieved from http://adventure.nationalgeographic.com/print/2008/08/everyday-survival/laurence-gonzales-text

they almost never do!), and who will freak out and become a potential liability? If I'm doing something that is risky, or if I'm a novice, I always make sure that I'm surrounded by people who I know can "be cool."

This saved me the first time I went on my first real rock-climbing trip. My boyfriend had invited me to climb the granite rock faces near Salt Lake City, and although I'd spent a few hours in a rock-climbing gym, I was new to the real thing. Overestimating my abilities, I fell, hit my head, and needed rescue across a raging river. The experienced climbers I was with were able to immediately move in, perform first aid, and set up a complicated Tyrolean traverse across the river with me hooked to one of the climbers. There may be another survival tip in this story. Know your limits!

Being cool has another purpose for people who are living with long-term life challenges like pain. When you're in a short-term survival situation, staying cool can mean the difference between life and death. Often the steps to take to avoid perishing, although daunting, are clear. You know that your efforts will either save you or you will die in the not-too-distant future. This isn't the case when you live with chronic disease or pain. When extreme discomfort doesn't go away, and a person has to live with the possibility that it never will, being cool takes on an entirely new meaning. Being cool comes to mean that you can resist the societal pressure to constantly look outside yourself to fix your pain. It means that you can avoid being so desperate that you fall prey to every new cure peddled by profit-seeking salespeople, or well-intentioned friends. It means that you can access your inner wisdom, which is always there to guide you towards comfort. You are able to revel in the spaces between the hardship, when your body for whatever reason, decides to move into ease. Being cool means that you can wake up every day of your life and tell yourself, "Today the pain will not crush me." You can let the strong emotions that pain unleashes move through you and drift away without taking them too seriously. This version of being cool is a different animal, one that takes time to develop and diligence to maintain. It also changes your life.

This is how Anderson Cooper responded when he was asked how he handled the dangers of traveling to war-torn areas:

> I don't believe you should be ruled by fear in anything in your life. I don't like anything that scares me and prefer to face it head on and get over it. Anyone who says they're not scared is a fool or liar or both. I just don't want that fear in my stomach to be part of my life so I work hard to eliminate it.[50]

What I like about this quote is that he says he prefers to face his fears and get over them instead of taking on fear as a way of life. This is a mark of a resilient person. Fear is a normal reaction to danger and an emotion that helps keep us alive. It is only when you allow fear to, as Anderson says, sit in your stomach and be part of your life, that it becomes harmful.

Here is an irony that comes with living in modern society. With all of the creature comforts we have access to, the freedom to live without being enslaved, modern conveniences that make our life much easier, we are more fearful than ever. Fear dominates political rhetoric and is subtly ingrained in mainstream media. Fear allows us to be manipulated, and once fears become deep-seated they move from the conscious mind into the subconscious mind where they turn into irrational beliefs.

"Fear," Shirley McClain has said, "is the most powerful weapon of mass destruction."[51] The reason that people who live in modern society are so fearful is because most of us have never really had to go to a place of real fear, the place where you have to decide whether to curl up in a corner and die or face your fears and move through them. This is where chronic disease can be a huge teacher; living with chronic disease brings with it much to fear: pain, disability, dependence, death, loss and lack, isolation, and abandonment. However, chronic disease also brings the opportunity to understand that even if all of these things happen to us, we can still choose to live with resilience.

---

[50]Keyes, C. (2010, March 08). Anderson Cooper: The Full Interview. Retrieved from http://www.outsideonline.com/1827816/anderson-cooper-full-interview

[51] MacLaine, S. (2011). *I'm over all that: And other confessions* (p. 6). New York: Atria Books.

"Only to the extent that we expose ourselves over and over to annihilation can that which is indestructible in us be found."
–Pema Chodron[52]

In order for anyone to understand just how strong they are, they have to be annihilated a bit first. Only then can they stand up, brush themselves off, and say, "If I can survive that I can survive anything." They can finally begin to understand that really, most of their fears are unfounded. The reality is that we are born with only two hard-wired fears: fear of loud noises and fear of heights. Every other fear we come up with has been learned, such as some of the most common fears of our modern age: flying, public speaking, intimacy, death, rejection, failure, and commitment. Fear blocks healing because it is rooted in lack of trust, the inability to believe that you are taken care of even during the most dire of situations, that you are always okay. Fear keeps you stuck in unhealthy relationships, dead-end jobs, and prevents you from trying to live the life you really want. Everyone I know, myself included, has at least one fear that prevents them from being a full expression of themselves. It is important to ask yourself fairly regularly, "What am I afraid of?" When you find your answer keep asking yourself "Why? Why am I afraid of this?" Often the answer will uncover deep-seated beliefs that came from your family, society, or partners, and have nothing to do with the truth.

Another question that can be helpful to ask yourself is, "What is the worst thing that can happen if what I'm afraid of actually comes to pass?" Whenever I've asked myself this I've realized that even the worst-case scenario is one that I can handle. Over the years I've thought, "What if I never get rid of my pain? "What if it stays with me forever?" This helped me to realize that even though I've lived with daily pain since age two, my life has been amazing on many levels. If I have to live the next forty-two years in pain I know I can do this, and I can still have a life that I will be grateful for.

Sometimes fears will stick. Fear of public speaking, for example, is one that many people will never get over. When fears stick, it is helpful to be honest with yourself and others about your fear. Acknowledge the fear isn't real, that you won't

---

[52] Chodron, P. (n.d.). DailyOM - When Things Fall Apart by Pema Chodron. Retrieved from http://www.dailyom.com/library/000/001/000001543.html

die from speaking in public even if you stutter the whole way through, and then give yourself some compassion. Nobody's perfect, after all. Over time you'll find that it is easier to become lighthearted, to even learn to laugh about your fear and it will never again dominate your life. Uncovering the truth of why you fear what you do is one of the most powerful things you can do to heal yourself and your life. Fear enslaves and the truth will set you free.

As I've gotten older and moved past my twenties and thirties, I've noticed something about my peers. At some point we all make a choice. We choose whether to become entrenched in our conditioning and settle into the life we've created for ourselves, or to make the effort to move beyond our conditioning and continue to learn and grow. I've observed people in the first category and inevitably I see them aging quicker, becoming more and more rigid in their thinking, less tolerant of others, and losing their ability to feel real joy. They are constantly stressed, running through their lives like hamsters on a wheel. The people in the latter category usually make big changes to their lifestyle at some point. They travel more, take classes, are better listeners, and have access to inner peace even if they aren't always feeling it. They look and act younger, and are much more adaptable in the ways that they live and think. I've come to understand that you cannot be resilient if you hold on to rigidity and stress.

A few years ago I was working as an occupational therapist at the Salt Lake City Veterans hospital. In so many ways I loved my job. I worked with wonderful, caring people, and had clients I liked and respected, some of whom became good friends. I learned a lot and had more opportunities there for learning than any job I'd ever had. The pay was good, and I didn't have to commute far. Why then, was I getting sick again? My body started to hurt at levels that were beyond a threshold that I could manage. My joints swelled up, and I had to steel myself every time I stood up from sitting, which became embarrassing when I'd have patients ask me, "Are you okay?" I was supposed to be asking them that. I continued to go to work every day, and suck it up as I've learned so well to do all my life. But then I had to say no to a trip with my parents that I'd been looking forward to for years. They invited me to go scuba diving in Palau, one of the best places to dive in the world, and I had to say no. I just couldn't physically do it. This was the last straw. There was absolutely no way I was going to let that happen again if I could help it. There had to be a way through this.

I began to think about what to do. At first the obvious came to mind: go to my doctor and find another drug to take. At the time I was taking an infusion drug that would last for about six months before I began to feel my joints start to swell again. But as I continued to weigh my options a question came to mind.

"What is the definition of insanity?" Doing the same thing over and over and expecting a different result. All my life I'd handled my flare-ups the exact same way. I'd become extremely upset, angry at myself, and frustrated by my fate. I'd look outside myself for answers about how to help myself, thinking that obviously I couldn't be trusted to do this since my body continued to betray me. I'd go to doctors, naturopaths, massage therapists, anyone who was around at the time, and I'd do what they told me. I thought about this and decided this time I was going to do things differently. Little did I know this decision would change my life. I ended up leaving all that was familiar to me, including how I thought. I realized that the only way I would ever become truly healthy was if I stopped being rigid. After all, if I wanted a more flexible body I couldn't have an inflexible mind.

Without rigid judgments cluttering my mind, I've been able to relax into my life and go with the flow more easily. Adaptability is the keystone to long-term resilience, because without it you will eventually get stuck. Once you challenge all your thoughts and break away from the ones that self-sabotage you'll be able to re-examine your life story. You can begin to stop seeing yourself as the victim, and start seeing yourself as the hero. There is nothing quite as redeeming as becoming your own hero.

"God, grant me the serenity to accept the things I cannot change, the courage to change the things I can, And the wisdom to know the difference." – The Serenity Prayer

Resilient people learn not to carry the world on their shoulders. They know that in order to stay sane they'll have to focus on what really matters to them, and stay away from ruminating about things that they have no control over. This way they can focus their energy on things that they can make a difference with, not things that will guarantee to continuously vex them.

There is another aspect to resilience that isn't talked about much: the ability to get out of survival mode as quickly as possible and stay out of survival mode whenever possible. Survival mode is how people deal with stress. Stress is triggered by the perception of threat. The actual definition of stress is, "The perception of physical or psychological threat and the perception that the individual's responses are inadequate to cope with that threat." Whenever a person feels stress, his or her body reacts by going into a fight-or-flight response. Physically this causes a cascade of bodily responses including a racing heart, release of glucose into the bloodstream, constriction of blood vessels to non-vital organs, increased muscle tension, and a deactivation of digestion and reproductive hormones. Because the fight-or-flight response isn't rational, it causes distorted thinking. When we are stressed it is easy to overreact to everything that happens to us, and see threats where they really don't exist. We can become stuck in survival mode, focusing on fear instead of love, and we end up closing our hearts and minds and limiting our possibilities.

I saw this a lot during my time at the Veterans Hospital. The men and women who spent time fighting foreign wars had to, by definition, spend most of their time abroad in survival mode, because if they didn't they would die. For months and years of their lives they learned how to keep themselves alive by being hyper-vigilant. However, once they got home and the threat was no longer there, they couldn't turn the stress off. Every single one of these people ended up with a stress-related illness. In fact, what I've noticed is that this is common to most veterans. When I first arrived at the Veterans Hospital I had just completed a week-long course on stress and mind-body healing, so the list of stress-related illnesses was fresh in my mind. As I looked at the medical record of each of my patients, I was surprised to see that every one of them had a condition on the list. Stress is a nemesis to resilience and a nemesis to health.

Many of us go through prolonged periods of severe stress, whether it's illness, a marriage break-up, the death of a loved one, or financial strain. One foundation to resilience is to be able to move through these periods without letting them suck you down the rabbit hole of stress. The best way to do this is to learn how to counteract stress in your body by doing activities that enable you to access inner peace and relaxation. The choices are many: meditation, prayer, deep breathing, yoga, chanting, exercising, or sitting in the tub. In fact, it's important to find methods that work for you and incorporate them into your daily life before heightened stress walks in and threatens to take over. You don't want to try learning to swim when you are about to sink.

"Someone was hurt before you, wronged before you, hungry before you, frightened before you, beaten before you, humiliated before you, raped before you ... yet, someone survived ... You can do anything you choose to do." – Maya Angelou[53]

I recently watched a movie called, *Love and Other Drugs*. It is a story about a cocky young drug rep, Jamie, who meets a beautiful young woman, Maggie, who has early onset Parkinson's disease, in a doctors' office where he is peddling his drugs. He is instantly enamored by her and they begin a passionate affair. She makes it clear that is all it will ever be, that she is not interested in a relationship. Being a young guy this is fine with him; as far as he is concerned he is living the dream. In spite of himself he falls for her and although she repeatedly pushes him away, eventually they end up together. She wants him only to see a sexy, beautiful, fun-loving person, and not the shaky, infirm side of her that is her disease, so whenever her disease takes hold she kicks him to the curb. Maggie is convinced that he won't want to be with her long-term when he could have any woman, especially the healthy version. So she keeps up the front for as long as she can, distracting him with juicy sex and a free-spirited attitude.

As far as Maggie is concerned, eventually she won't be able to be wild and free; she'll most likely be old and slowly dying at the age of thirty, just when her peers are getting married and starting a family. She might as well soak up life while she can, have the experiences that will keep her smiling when she begins to lose the ability to care for herself. She's decided to have flings with beautiful men, keep them all at arms length and let them go before they see the less attractive side of her. Maggie is protecting herself from being devastated by the fact that no man would want to be with a beautiful, yet doomed woman. Parkinson's is hell, she would give anything to run away from it forever, so there is no way she would blame any man for doing the same. At one point in the movie Jamie meets

---

[53] T, V. (n.d.). Someone was hurt before you... Retrieved from
http://www.wisdomcommons.org/wisbits/4693-someone-was-hurt-before-you

a man whose wife has the disease. Jamie asks for advice and the man told him to pack his bags, saying that MS isn't a disease, it is a Russian novel.

The movie has the typical Hollywood happy ending. Jamie chooses to be with Maggie and she chooses to let him in. Don't we all wish that life would be like the movies? Reality, though, sometimes can suck. Here are some statistics:

- Divorce rates among people where one spouse is chronically ill are over 75%.[54]

- Divorce rates for people with rheumatoid arthritis are 70% higher than that of the general population (American Journal of Medicine) and people with RA are five times less likely to remarry than people with osteoarthritis (a much less severe disease) [55]

- A 2009 study published in the journal Cancer looked at 515 people who had brain tumors, cancer, or multiple sclerosis and were married at the time of their diagnosis. After six months 11.6 % of the couples were separated or divorced. Here is where it gets interesting; if the woman was the one with the illness the rate of break-up was 20%, if the man was the person with the illness, the rate was 2.9%. 96% of the breakups among people with multiple sclerosis were among couples where the one with the disease was the wife. The fact is that a woman is six times more likely to end up separated or divorced soon after a diagnosis of cancer or MS than a man who becomes ill with the same disease.[56]

Sometimes Hollywood movies, despite themselves, contain pearls of wisdom. Chronic disease is a Russian novel. When I watched the movie, I related all too well to Maggie. I've spent most of my life, as I tell myself, avoiding the inevitable, dating men I knew would never have the strength to handle my disease, so when we parted ways I wouldn't be emotionally destroyed. I have worked to stay open while hoping deep down

[54] Sifferlin, A. (2014, May 1). Till death do us part-unless it's the wife who gets sick. Retrieved from http://time.com/83486/divorce-is-more-likely-if-the-wife-not-the-husband-gets-sick/
[55] Young, K. (2012, May 29). Is Rheumatoid Arthritis a Factor in Divorce? Retrieved from http://rawarrior.com/is-rheumatoid-arthritis-a-factor-in-divorce/
[56] Parker-Pope, T. (2009, November 12). Divorce Risk Higher When Wife Gets Sick. Retrieved from http://well.blogs.nytimes.com/2009/11/12/men-more-likely-to-leave-spouse-with-cancer/?_r=0

one day to meet someone strong enough to take me on, but I know that the odds are slim. Knowing that love, sex, support, partnership, and connection are all things that keep one healthy, and are beautiful gifts that life has to offer, I also know that I may have to miss out because of my disease. The truth is, I'm still waiting, hoping, and staying open. As far as I'm concerned, if I'm going to be in a committed relationship I'm going to be someone who defies the odds or I'm not going to play the game at all.

Resilience means that you have to look at your life with clear eyes and acknowledge the reality of your situation. Let go of what you think your life should look like and instead accept what is. This doesn't mean that you give up on your dreams or give in to a sad fate. It doesn't mean that you stop seeking true connection and keeping your heart open to love and life. Resilient people know that sometimes the odds are long, but they never stop trying. They never stop living the life they want within the parameters of the hand they were dealt.

When I first read the statistics about chronic disease and divorce I had to ask, "Why? Why would men and woman so readily give up on their vows to their spouse, the person they chose to spend the rest of their life with?" There are the obvious answers: they stop being attracted to their partner, they become so exhausted they couldn't do it anymore, the relationship died because they felt like caregivers instead of lovers, their spouse became too much of a financial drain. These are just excuses. The real answer is that they've stopped being resilient. They've given into fear. They've stopped being honest with themselves and their spouse. They move towards denial as a state of being. I'll admit that maybe they never were honest, and in this case the marriage would eventually break down regardless. But the people faced with chronic disease in a marriage who have lost the ability to bounce back from challenge and hardship need to recover their resilience.

"We cannot change the cards we were dealt, just how we play the hand." –Randy Pausch[57]

There is something to be said for sucking the juice out of life while you can, stretching the boundaries of what you think you are capable of. Moving out of your comfort zone. Throwing

---

[57] Randy Pausch. (n.d.). Retrieved from http://en.wikiquote.org/wiki/Randy_Pausch

caution to the wind. Being brave in your choices. Deciding to do it now, because you don't know if and when you'll ever get the chance again.

People often give me a hard time for what they perceive as me pushing myself too hard when, for example, I take a long bike ride, scuba dive twice, and go out dancing in one day. But for me, this day may be the last one in a long while that I'll be able to be this carefree. Days like this are days that I'll never forget and never regret. This is my reality, one that only I truly know and only I will experience.

Those around me who are bound to me by love live vicariously with the pain and the accomplishment that my disease brings. The people who choose to see me with clear eyes will begin to understand and accept that my situation isn't ideal, it perhaps isn't one that anyone would choose, but it is my life. And as a resilient person I choose to find joy and hope in all that I experience. When all else fails, I look at my situation with all the curiosity I can muster and I say, "Hmm, isn't this interesting!" and I try to laugh. I've learned that the people I can truly let in are the ones who can laugh with me.

Any victory worth something comes with pain, a taste or two of failure, and is hard won. Knowing this going in helps to soothe the soul when you feel like you are lost in the ocean of life, treading water but not getting anywhere. Resilient people understand that the one and only way toward having the life they want is to keep trying, and, like Winston Churchill, they never, never, never give up. They are adept at transforming fear of failure and negativity and using these things as fuel to drive them to success. They see challenges as opportunities to gain strength and life skills that will help them be better people in the long run. And through it all they keep their focus on peace of mind, the inner calm underneath the storms that life can bring – the peace of mind that can come from following Immanuel Kant's Rules for Happiness: Something to do, Someone to love, and Something to hope for. It's as easy and as hard as that.

SELF-CARE

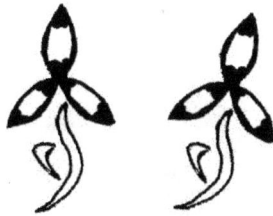

"The body says what words cannot."
– Martha Graham[58]

---

[58] Martha Graham Reflects on Her Art and a Life in Dance. (1985, March 31). Retrieved from http://partners.nytimes.com/library/arts/033185graham.html

Our bodies can be a source of great pleasure and unbearable pain. We are each given one body to take us through our life and once we are born there is no escaping. We see, hear, feel, and touch every second of every day of our lives. We experience our environment through the filter of our body and create thoughts around this experience that shape our reality.

For most of my life physical pain has tainted my filter. Pain has made my movement hesitant and drained me of the energy my body creates to carry me through the day. As a youngster, pain prevented me from feeling truly carefree. I've always felt a tinge of envy when I see people demonstrating physical prowess that I know I'll never have: running, climbing, jumping across rocks on a river, skating on ice – these are activities that are often too difficult because of my pain. My feelings of envy, however, don't hold a candle to the shame and loathing I've felt when I've compared myself to others and to my own idea of who I should be. Over the years I've felt shame in so many things: my crooked fingers and toes, my arm that is two inches shorter than the other, my limp, my swollen knees, my difficulty with kneeling and squatting.

Finally I realized that waking up with pain and feeling dismay at my swollen knees was not a good way to start the day. Having pain and joint swelling does limit me, but the real limits, I've discovered, are self-imposed. These limits are the ones I've placed on myself because of how I've felt about myself. For example, I have sometimes chosen not to wear rings that I like because I don't want people looking at my hands. I have said no to tubing on the river because I don't want my difficulty with getting in and out of the water to be seen. "What if," I thought, "I lived to the fullest within my limits instead of narrowing my experiences even more because of how I felt about them?" This thought began to transform the way I experienced the world by shifting my relationship to my body.

The first thing I did was begin to notice my thoughts and how they influenced my actions. If I decided not to wear my favorite short skirt because I wanted to hide my swollen knees, I'd observe this. Then I'd casually ask my friends if they were aware of how my knees looked. I was shocked when they had to look closely before they saw what to me were embarrassingly huge knees. The truth is that most people are too wrapped up in their own imagined imperfections to notice yours. It's funny, really, if you think about it. Next time you're at the beach and feeling self-conscious about how you look in a bathing suit, look around and ask yourself how many people are feeling the same way. I'd venture a guess that at least 95% of the people over ten years of age are in the same boat.

To a large degree the level of comfort or discomfort we feel in our bodies is directly influenced by how we feel about our bodies – our self-image. Instead of being captive to a negative self-image and living in a self-imposed cage, why not decide to be your own best friend? The one who tells you how sweet you look in your favorite dress and means it? Who revels in your accomplishments and cheers you on as you change unhealthy habits? The friend who is always there to tell you how wonderful you are when you are feeling less than desirable?

Before you can ever take positive action on behalf of yourself, you have to see yourself as someone who deserves what you are seeking. You have to believe that you are worth it, deep in your core, not just at the level of lip-service. You have to love yourself, warts and all.

"Compassion for oneself is the greatest healer of all."
–Anonymous

A few years ago I decided to see a psychologist who specialized in working with people in pain. One day he told me, "Studies show that people who accept their pain do better than those who don't." Until then I had really enjoyed our time together, but in my view there were so many things wrong with that sentence I didn't know what to say. First of all, any sentence that begins with "Studies show ..." in reference to me won't hold my attention. Secondly, in my opinion, accepting pain is an oxymoron. "Why in the world would I want to accept my pain?" I thought. I couldn't come up with a single thing acceptable about it. "What were those accepting people doing better at?" I wondered. It took me a long time to come to terms with his statement, and when I did it was because I had decided to make peace with my body and come up with my own version of acceptance. I decided it was okay to not accept a life of pain as long as I accepted the present moment, which may involve pain. I can accept the pain I feel right now while at the same time hoping that tomorrow will feel better. And most important, I can learn to look at my swollen knees with love and compassion, understanding that they are trying their hardest to perform for me. It's easy to love your body when it feels good, but loving it when it doesn't is true love. Love your body without limits and you'll see your life begin to expand, because your relationship with the world is a reflection of your relationship with yourself.

When I turned thirty-three I thought it was my lucky year. At the time I had just moved to Morro Bay, on the central coast of California. I was dating a new man who was caring, kind, and really wanted to know how I felt, which considering my past dating history up to that point was a miracle. I had a job that I didn't like very much, but the hours were good and it paid well. The arthritis had been in remission for about three years at that time. Life was smooth sailing. Then my beautiful house of cards started to crumble.

The first sign was a change in my body. The arthritis started to talk to me again. In the beginning it was subtle enough to be nothing more than an annoying bother, but soon the symptoms began to grow. A swollen knee, a painful elbow, a sore ankle in the morning; it's amazing what I was able to push aside until the monkey on my back became a gorilla. One day I woke up and had a hard time lifting the down comforter off my body because it hurt so much and I knew I was in trouble. I soon found myself at the doctor getting pumped full of steroids through an IV. Looking back, the path leading to the longest, most intense, and scariest flare-up of my life wasn't hard to follow.

A year earlier I was living in Pagosa Springs, Colorado. Being single in a small town is always an interesting experience, especially because of the one-degree-of-separation rule. Before you meet anyone new, you probably already know him or her through a friend. So when I met Jim at a party and gave him my number, I'd heard about his past dating history from my roommate and I had been to the restaurant he owned. I'd even had a conversation with one of his employees, a motherly woman who remarked to me, "Poor Jim is so sad about breaking up with his girlfriend that he hasn't been himself. Are you available?" (At the time I wasn't.) He'd also recently been a patient at the clinic where I worked. Knowing him vicariously meant that when we went on our first date my guard was down a bit. Maybe because he was older and appeared wiser I was easily influenced by him. When he strongly suggested that I go on birth control pills before we started having sex and offered to drive me to Planned Parenthood, I readily agreed despite the fact that I'd been wary of the pill all my life and had had a bad experience the one time I'd taken it in the past. After a few weeks taking this new drug I began to have bad stomachaches, unbearable itchy rashes, and in general didn't feel very good. Despite this I kept up with Jim doing the long mountain bike rides he enjoyed, drinking margaritas, and sleeping too little. This was my first set of mistakes.

After a few months I finally broke down and went to an allergist. When I told him that birth control pills were the only new drug I was taking he said, "They won't cause an allergy, it must be something else." But instead of trying to find out what that something else was, he gave me prednisone. Prednisone is a powerful steroid medication that works wonders for allergic reactions and controlling inflammation, but it also has extremely negative side effects, so people only use it long term if there is no other option. A few months later I moved to California and I knew that I had to do something. By this time I trusted myself enough to question what the doctor had told me. I took myself off the pill and the prednisone. (A word of caution: Please never do this without a doctor advising you, because prednisone is such a strong drug it causes the adrenal glands to atrophy. If you don't wean yourself off of it slowly you can go into something called adrenal crisis.) Lo and behold, I felt just fine!

Moving from Colorado had been stressful. I knew I needed to leave but wasn't sure where I was going to go. I pressured myself to find a place to live and a job right away and worked hard to make this happen. By the time I landed in California I was exhausted, but I pushed myself to dive into my new life with fervor. On the surface it appeared that I had successfully created the life that I wanted. I worked at a rehabilitation hospital and spent my free time biking, hiking, meeting new friends, and spending time with my boyfriend who I'd met when I first arrived in town. There was something missing though, and by the time I realized what it was I was too far down the rabbit hole to get out. In the midst of creating my successful life, I'd forgotten to honor the most important relationship of my life. I'd forgotten to take care of myself.

"Our bodies are our gardens to which our wills are gardeners."
–William Shakespeare[59]

Each of us goes through life with a jumble of contradictory motives. These motives guide our behavior and shape our lives. Many motives are easy to identify and explain. The desire for success and the need to feel useful, loved, caring, and cared-for are all motives that most of us share. Early on in life we are taught what success, being useful, caring, and feeling loved look like, and this influences our behavior throughout life. We also have hidden motives that stem from our need to be true to ourselves. These desires may not be as socially acceptable, especially in the family we grow up in.

Like many people I was taught that success involved accomplishing a lot, going to the best college and university, getting a good job and working full-time. The way towards happiness was to keep busy with an active social life, spending time with like-minded people to share my experiences, and to never open up when I was feeling less than fine. Caring for others meant that I put their needs before my own and worked hard to never be a burden.

There were a few problems with this. My body didn't have the energy it took to prove I was "happy." I actually liked spending time with people who were much different from me; it satisfied my natural curiosity. I inherently have itchy feet which means that I'm a natural nomad and no good at staying with one job for more than a few years. The intense pain that I felt on a daily basis made my life a challenge, which I was unable to share with those around me. For most of my life I hid my desires and my hidden motives from everyone, including myself.

My assumed motives were showing me one way to navigate life, and my internal compass was calling me somewhere else entirely. So I spent years conflicted, beating down my hidden motives with a metaphorical stick. The self-harm I was doing, however, wasn't so metaphorical. Whenever my body became so exhausted I could barely see straight, I would berate myself and begrudgingly rest for the minimum time required. I would fight through pain as if my life depended on it, hiking with

---

[59] No Fear Shakespeare: Othello: Act1, Scene 3, Page 13. (n.d.). Retrieved from http://nfs.sparknotes.com/othello/page_52.html

bleeding blisters that I barely acknowledged and strapping ace bandages to my sore knees so that I could keep going at work. Whenever asked how I was feeling I said "fine" even if this wasn't really true. In living up to the motives that were handed down to me as a child, I was inflicting harm on myself.

One day I was watching the movie *Good Will Hunting*, which features Matt Damon as Will Hunting, a young math savant working as a janitor at Harvard. Will grew up in foster homes, was beaten as a kid, and told he was worthless. He found himself repeatedly in court for fighting and burglary, always able to talk himself out of jail because he was so smart. In the movie Will gets into yet another fight, and this time the judge orders him to be tutored in math by Harvard professors and go to counseling. He sees a psychologist, Sean McGuire, played by Robin Williams, who also grew up on the "wrong side of the tracks," and who actually understands where he's coming from. He sees his hidden motives, his internal compass. Sean knows that fighting is Will's way of trying to hurt himself, because he thinks he deserves it. He thinks the treatment he received as a young kid is his fault. One day Sean shows him pictures taken of his bruised body by social workers while he was in foster care and he says, "It's not your fault." Will looks embarrassed and replies, "I know." Sean repeats, "It's not your fault." Will says, "Yeah, I know." Sean keeps repeating, "It's not your fault. It's not your fault," until Will gets angry and breaks down crying. Watching the movie I started bawling with him. I suddenly realized that all the years I had spent berating myself for needing rest, ignoring my pain, I was blaming myself. Deep down I thought it was my fault. Obviously having arthritis meant that there was something wrong with me; somewhere inside I had twisted myself into thinking that there must be something wrong with me so I was given this disease. I hated my disease, I blamed myself, and so I hurt myself.

Years went by before I understood that until I could uncover all of my motives, and see myself with clear eyes, I would never be healthy. I needed to make peace with the warring forces of my head and heart. I needed to practice self-wisdom, not self-betrayal. Before you can take care of yourself you need to know who you are. And you need to honor that knowledge.

In the book *The Biology of Belief*, cell biologist Bruce Lipton explains how we are programmed at a young age to interact with the world. Very early on in our life we are subtly taught how to think, feel, and act. Some people claim this starts before birth, but it is clear from brain imaging studies that beginning at birth we are putty in the hands of our parents. Human beings have evolved to value experiential learning (nurture) over preprogrammed behavior (nature). The instincts that humans are born with, such as the ability to swim and hold our breath under water, all have plasticity, meaning that they can easily be overridden through learned behavior. How many people develop a fear of water when their parents are overzealous about keeping them away from it because they are afraid their child will drown?

The adult brain functions with a variety of brainwave patterns depending on what is required. The lowest EEG frequency is called Delta, and in adults this is associated with deep sleep and healing. From birth to the age of two, the infant's brain is operating mostly at the level of Delta. At age two this pattern shifts into Theta, a brainwave associated with meditation and relaxation, creativity, day-dreaming, and deep emotion. These two brainwaves keep an individual in a highly suggestible state, which is how young children can learn an immense amount of information about how to behave and what to think. We acquire the beliefs and behaviors that our parents teach us through this subconscious programming, enabled by these brainwaves. In fact, hypnotherapy is so effective because it accesses the brain by putting subjects into Theta/Delta states. Hypnotherapy can uncover the motives that are driving our behavior and reprogram our subconscious mind to behave in a more healthy manner.

Consider the depth and breadth of each person's parental learning. In this life-learning soup there are great tools for living well, such as the need to eat your vegetables, but you may also have taken on your mother's fear of being fat and emotional eating patterns. If as a child you sat at the dinner table, which modeled a balanced meal, but also observed your Mom sneaking cookies on the ride home from soccer practice, you were receiving mixed messages about food that will influence your behavior as an adult. Even worse, if your Mom limited your intake and emphasized the horrors of sugar, you would most likely carry that fear with you and end up conflicted as you battled internally with hunger cues and an innate fondness for sweet foods.

Most of us have ten healthy beliefs and habits for each unhealthy one but one unhealthy belief can become the driving force of your life, derailing you if you don't weed it out of the garden of your mind. As I mentioned earlier, for me this one unhealthy belief was that somehow the arthritis was my fault. Because of this skewed idea I spent most of my young years trying to hide it from my peers. I'm sure there were a few people who wondered about how many "sprained ankles" I had when I was in junior high school. It also caused me to adopt a no-pain-no-gain attitude. If this was my lot in life, if I had somehow created this, I'd better just learn to suck it up. Where did this crazy belief come from? Why would a young child blame herself for having a disease that she had no hand in creating? I didn't have wicked parents who told me this. I didn't have a Dr. Strangelove whispering evil nothings into my ear. If there had, it would have been easy to pinpoint the source of my misery. No, my self-torture had a more subtle cause. I was a sensitive, curious child, who didn't want to be a bother. I heard my parents always insist how well I was doing to those around them even when I was in intense pain. I paid attention when they enrolled me in tennis, swimming, softball, and summer camp despite my small size and pain. The more I heard this as a youngster, the more I thought it had to be true, and I began to doubt myself.

When I was in the seventh grade we received a call from a major news station in New York City. They were doing a story on rheumatoid arthritis and had gotten my name from my doctor. They wanted to send their top anchorwoman, Michelle Marsh, to our house to interview my parents and I about what it was like to live with rheumatoid arthritis. I was excited about the attention and began to think about what I would say. Would I tell them that I wore splints at night that usually ended up across the room in the morning because I'd take them off and throw them in my sleep? Would I tell them how tiring it was? Could I admit to how lonely and scared I felt when I'd see other kids playing in the park with glee? In the end none of this mattered, because when Michelle Marsh and her film crew got there they began talking to my father. "How well does Kathryn function at home?" she asked my Dad, who quickly replied, "She does great, just great. Her Mom exercises her joints in the morning before school and after that she has no problem at all!" Too bad that wasn't true. I was taken aback and decided not to contradict him.

My Dad mentioned that I was on the school basketball team, neglecting to say that I was the bench warmer and would only play when the team was thirty points ahead. The film crew took me out to the backyard and proceeded to film me shooting baskets. I was mortified. Then I had the thought that the kids in school may end up seeing the show and I became even more embarrassed. To my relief, my brief brush with fame came to a sudden halt when the station decided not to air my part. Apparently, they had already decided to paint a different picture of rheumatoid arthritis, so they aired a segment featuring a woman who complained she was too depressed to get out of bed most mornings. This episode taught me two things: the media has an agenda that has more to do with ratings than truth, and the adults around me didn't see my truth.

Over time, this led me to trust other people's opinions about me over my own. I gave my power away to doctors, loved ones, boyfriends, and even the occasional salesperson. When you don't trust yourself, your identity shrinks until you become nothing but a reflection of those around you. I had to almost disappear before the shift back to self-regard began and it took many years before I could truly say that I no longer betrayed my own wisdom on a regular basis.

Self-care is a natural extension of self-regard, but even for people with rock-solid self-regard it can still take time to build into your life. Weeding through the mire of information about health that bombards us can be daunting and overwhelming. Has anyone else noticed just how contradictory "expert" advice can be? As an experiment I did an Internet search. The first one was, "health benefits of coconut oil." I found a long list including: hair care; skin care, stress relief, maintaining cholesterol levels, weight loss, increased immunity, proper digestion and metabolism, relief from kidney problems, heart disease, high blood pressure, diabetes, HIV and cancer, dental care, and bone strength. Then I modified the search to, "health risks of coconut oil." There I found this statement from Livestrong.com: "Coconut oil is a saturated fat. This fat is linked to the development of numerous serious diseases, including heart disease, high cholesterol, obesity, and diabetes complications."

What is a person supposed to make of this contradictory information? High-protein diet, low-protein diet, six hours sleep or ten hours, low-intensity exercise or high-intensity; Google any of these items and you'll find advocates for and those who have dire warnings against. If it weren't so important to know, it would be comical. Whenever there is a new health fad in medicine I sit back and wait for the backlash that will inevitably occur. Vitamin E was touted as vital in arthritis treatment until it was vilified after a John Hopkins study that showed supplementing with more than 400 IUs per day increased risk of death. Now vitamin D is the new wonder vitamin. I've decided that what works for me is to spend time in the sun every day and call it good.

Over the years I've changed my health habits because of advice from chiropractors, naturopathic doctors, acupuncturists, MDs, massage therapists, and many others whom I've consulted to help me with the rheumatoid arthritis. Each of these well-meaning professionals has educated me about their point of view and what they feel is the best way to improve my health. My doctor will tell me that I have an overactive immune system and that I need to suppress it so that it doesn't destroy my joints. My acupuncturist will tell me that I have a damp condition, blocked chi, and I need to balance my meridians. The naturopathic doctor will tell me my problems originate with my digestion and that I need to eliminate most foods from my diet until I detox, and my massage therapist will tell me that stimulating my lymph flow will move the swelling from my joints. The truth is that at times all of them and none of them have been correct.

Self-care is learning what your body needs to function well and respecting it enough to give it those things. How many hours of sleep do you need? If you can't answer this question, it is time to find out. Whenever you can, sleep until you wake up naturally, until you have an understanding of what your natural sleep rhythm is. What kinds of exercise do you respond best to? What foods work well for you? When answering these questions it's important to tune into your own inner guidance and forget what you think the answers should be. Looking outward for answers about diet, exercise, or sleep is helpful for general guidance, but in the end it is important to ask yourself what is true for you. And keep asking, because over time the answers will change.

"The amount of sleep required by the average person is five minutes more." –Wilson Mizner[60]

Sleep, like health, is an activity that we all take for granted until we don't get enough. Sometimes sleep deprivation is caused by busy lives, but when sleep becomes difficult without cause, nighttime is a long and torturous event. In fact, sleep deprivation is one of the oldest forms of torture. The ancient Romans termed it "tormentum vigilae," or waking torture. Scientists are still debating why we need sleep, but no one's debating just how awful a person feels when they don't get enough. If you have difficulty sleeping, you are in good company; up to 75% of Americans say they have sleeping problems. People are getting 20% less sleep than they did a century ago, and to rectify this they hanker for pills. Prescriptions for sleeping pills are sharply increasing worldwide. In the U.S. alone, doctors wrote 60 million prescriptions for sleeping pills in 2010. Sleep is vitally important for self-care and necessary for maintaining performance in concentration, forming memories, self-healing, and brain function.

I've always loved to sleep. To me it's like taking a trip and not knowing where you're going to end up. Dreaming takes me to different places every night, helps me to sort through difficult emotions, and always entertains me in the morning. Sleep gives me an excuse to rest for an extended period every day. How much harder I would push myself if I didn't sleep? How endless would life feel? Unfortunately, sleep for me at times is so elusive it is frightening. I've spent endless hours lying in bed, with nowhere to go but the dark recesses of my mind, anxiety seeping into my pores and helping to perpetuate my sleepless state. Over time, the necessity of my need for sleep became the mother of my inventing ways to help myself to do this. I consulted sleep experts, did my own research, tried many things, and eventually found what works for me.

The first thing I found out is how much sleep I need to feel rested. My magic number is eight to nine hours. Then I developed a sleep routine that works for me. Experts will tell people with sleep issues not to do anything in bed but sleep and sex, but for me reading in bed relaxes me and removes most of

---

[60] Wilson Mizner Quote. (n.d.). Retrieved from http://www.azquotes.com/quote/579747

the pre-sleep anxiety that I may feel. I keep the bedroom cool, but not cold, and have a fan for white noise. Earplugs have been my best friend at times and so has my mp3 player. After discovering brainwave therapy, which uses sound waves to synchronize your brainwaves into delta, the brainwave your body moves into during deep sleep, I've never left home without it. During the rare occasions when my body decides not to sleep, brainwave therapy has literally saved my sanity. I never look at the clock when I can't sleep and have learned how to relax my mind even when sleep isn't coming by reminding myself just how resilient I am. Over the years I've tried so many different herbal regimes for sleep that naming them would fill a small book. Over time I've learned which ones work best for me and how to rotate them so I never get dependent on any one thing. I've managed to steer clear of prescription drugs, although Benadryl has traveled with me quite a bit.

I know people who sleep best with music playing and others who swear by warm milk. Despite what you read or hear about the do's and don'ts of good sleep, you know your body best. If you feel comfortable doing something that defies all logical reasoning, go for it as long as you know this is enhancing your sleep. Sleep is a conditioned response, meaning it responds to specific stimuli, or behaviors. If chocolate milk is the stimulus your body responds well to, there is no reason to stop using this even if experts advise against chocolate at night.

Sleep can be your friend, not your enemy. Despite any sleep issues you may have, quality, restful sleep is not out of your grasp. Make this a priority and you'll be amazed at the changes you will see.

"A man's health can be judged by which he takes two at a time – pills or stairs." –Joan Welsh[61]

Modern society has created an unusual lifestyle that to our knowledge has never before appeared in human history. Exercise is no longer a by-product of moving through your day; it has morphed into a separate activity that has to be planned. We have also invented more types of exercise than ever before. Pilates, Zumba, shake weights, and pole dancing are all creative

---

[61] Joan Welsh (1958-) American Blogger, Writer, Journalist Anderson, C. H. (2012, January 3). The Smartest Things Ever Said About Fitness. Retrieved from http://www.shape.com/fitness/workouts/smartest-things-ever-said-about-fitness/slide/7

activities that are the result of our sedentary lifestyle. So are modern diseases including metabolic syndrome, diabetes type 2, heart disease, and osteoporosis.

A healthy life has to include exercise; there are no exceptions. The question isn't whether you need to, it's what do you need to do. People approach exercise in a myriad of ways. For some people getting exercise over as quickly as possible is the goal. I have a friend who is in a self-proclaimed, "run to drink beer" club; he chooses running because, as he said, "You don't have to run as long in order to get a good workout." For others, exercise is an enjoyable activity that they look forward to and miss if they don't get regularly. Luckily for me, I'm in the latter category.

When I was thirty-four, the rheumatoid arthritis flared badly. One way that I knew I was really in trouble was when I saw bikers on the road and didn't feel a twinge of envy; I only felt tired. At the time, I got out daily and walked on the beach. I would wrap my knees and ankles in ace bandages and walk for as long as I could, which sometimes was only ten minutes, sit and rest, and then keep going. Walking helped me bear the sadness of my circumstance and helped me to feel more in control. There have also been times when my swelling and pain changed dramatically on a daily basis. This situation made planning exercise very hard. How could I commit to a yoga class when it was extremely likely that on the day of the class my knees would look like grapefruits? So I decided to chuck out any preconceived notions about what I would do on a particular day and decided to move my body every day. Some days my body wanted to do a five-mile hike, and other days a twenty-minute walk sufficed.

I think that for many people exercise becomes an overwhelming task because they set high exercise goals. Then they wind up failing to reach their goals, allow their self-esteem to take a hit, and give up entirely. If only they would have decided to move their body every day and set parameters for what that movement would look like. Physical prowess is one of the delights of being human and one of my secret pet peeves is when I see able-bodied people who squander their physical potential, potential that I would cherish like the most precious stone if I had it. Honor the body with exercise and it will honor you back with improved health.

"Let your food be your medicine and your medicine be your food." -Hippocrates.[62]

Hippocrates also said, "If we could give every individual the right amount of nourishment and exercise, not too little and not too much, we would have found the safest way to health."[63] Smart man. Any journey towards health will eventually lead to nutrition, and when it does confusion will inevitably set in. Researching healthy diets one will encounter a mire of often conflicting advice. Eat grains, or avoid them like the plague; it's difficult to decide. The food industry will be happy to help as they are masters at molding what we eat and the way we eat it.

This era of improved nutritional knowledge has served to muddy the waters even more. Although there are definite links to food consumption and health, as well as ill-health, there is no definitive answer about who should eat what. As complicated as nutrition science has become, in my opinion the truth is simple, and the simple truth is that eating a variety of real food, and not too much is the basis for a healthy diet.

Being healthy from the inside-out is more than that. It also involves eating with a good attitude. Healthy eating is done with enjoyment, appreciation, and pleasure as well as good sense. Sadly, for many of us eating has become associated with guilt, fear, and poor body image. How many times have you witnessed someone eating a large dessert while exclaiming, "This is SO bad, I really shouldn't." "If you shouldn't, then don't," I want to say, "but if you are eating a yummy dessert, for goodness sakes, enjoy it!" Food is tied to body image, self-esteem, and self-control. The fact that sixty-five percent of women in the United States and almost one million men suffer from an eating disorder is a sad reflection of our relationships to ourselves.

My relationship to food and eating has changed dramatically over the years. After a typical childhood where eating was done three times a day and occasional goodies were allowed, I became a pre-teen who developed anorexia. Food became

[62] Hippocrates (c. 460 bc -c. 375) A Greek Physician in the Classical period, a contemporary of Aristotle and Plato, is considered the father of modern medicine. He is known for his medical writings, being a great physician and teacher, and for influencing the ethics of medicine, (The Hippocratic Oath). He was called by his contemporaries the "Great Physician."
[63] "Hippocrates Quote." BrainyQuote. Xplore, n.d. Web. 29 May 2015.

something I limited as much as possible. I ate only enough to keep alive and no more, which eventually landed me in a hospital when it became obvious to my doctors that I wasn't doing a good enough job. Looking back, anorexia was almost an unavoidable issue. I had parents who were hyper-aware of weight, especially in my older sister who was never rail thin like me. I observed as they encouraged her to go on diets and how they watched her eating like a hawk. I was a "good girl" who never got in trouble and was always trying to please my elders. I was sensitive to criticism, emotionally inhibited, intelligent, and deep down I blamed myself for my arthritis.

It began when I was fourteen. I began to menstruate and the second period I experienced didn't stop. To make life even more exciting, I was on a week-long skiing vacation with three families at the time and ended up having my forehead cut open when a woman plowed into me. This threw me into the air, landing me sideways on her ski edge. I kept skiing, but as the week went by I got more and more tired, not knowing that going through a whole box of maxi-pads in a day was not normal. The end result of this was five days in the hospital as they replaced my blood and gave me hormone pills. These hormone pills encouraged weight gain, which, along with normal puberty, gave me curves that I wasn't comfortable with.

So I stopped eating. This may seem hard, but in the scheme of things hunger is not so bad, especially when compared to chronic pain. And there was an amazing perk: When I starved myself long enough, the arthritis went away. I'm guessing that my body was too exhausted at that point to do anything but survive. During the next year I kept withering away, surprisingly right under the noses of my parents, and it wasn't until I was weighed during a doctor appointment that I was finally busted. I remember at the time being surprised at how easily the people around me were manipulated. Not having much practice at lying before this, it amazed me how naturally this dubious skill came to me. I lied about what I ate, how much, and who with every day. I'd push foods around my plate and tell my best friend Beth that I didn't need to eat because, unlike her, I wasn't playing on any sports teams. I did this until I was placed in the children's ward of Columbia Presbyterian Medical Center in New York City.

I think anorexia didn't kill me for two reasons. I have a strong will to live, and my doctor didn't strip away all my control by feeding me through an IV. Many other doctors were handling their young patients this way, and during my time in the Children's ward I saw a few of them struggle with being completely defeated. They all eventually disappeared.

I left the hospital after six months, but it took me many years to unravel my complicated feelings about this time of my life and to trust myself again. When I discovered healthy eating and began to experiment with different anti-inflammatory diets, part of me was concerned that this was a disguise for slipping back into an eating disorder, especially because it was always so easy. When you go to the extremes that I did to lose weight trying a gluten-free diet is a walk in the park. Once my willpower kicked in, I didn't have to think about it. For most people with juvenile arthritis, the barest possibility that altering diet could improve symptoms would be more than enough to give it a try. But what about for someone like me, who'd survived the most deadly mental illness, anorexia, which kills ten percent of its victims? Someone like me, who trusted other people's opinion more that my own when it came to my body?

I had to shift my complicated feelings about food before I could finally eat with an attitude that fostered health and wellbeing. I had to free myself from my past, and let go of any doubt that anorexia still wielded control over my actions. I had to have conversations with my parents about the anxiety they felt when I chose to change my diet and conversations with myself about what my true motivations were. I was able to rediscover the pleasure that food gave me before the anorexia took over, and steer my palate toward a life-giving, healing, flexible, way of eating.

Eat to please yourself and heal your body. Let others do the same and together enjoy one of the most pleasurable ways to health.

"The man who doesn't relax and hoot a few hoots voluntarily, now and then, is in great danger of hooting hoots and standing on his head for the edification of the pathologist and trained nurse, a little later on." –Elbert Hubbard[64]

Stress is the bane of modern existence; unless you learn how to manage your stress you will end up ill. Billions of dollars have

---

[64] Elbert Hubbard. (n.d.). Retrieved from http://izquotes.com/quote/290444

been spent treating stress-related illnesses, and many of us live a daily existence awash in it. The example that best helped me get a better perspective on stress comes from Willie Nelson, a man who hasn't wasted many learning opportunities in his life. In his book *The Tao of Willie*, he talks about what he calls The Willie Way. The Willie Way involves, among other things, taking his philosophy with a grain of salt, letting your anger go, stopping your excessive worry about what someone else is doing or saying, and stopping excessive worry in general. Volumes have been written about taming the mind, thousands of years of practice have been done by monks and laypeople, and here Willie, in his infinite wisdom, condenses it all down to this:

> Now if you want to go through life pissed off about traffic and jackasses, that's your business, but do so at the risk of not noticing the other driver who kindly let you in when your lane ended, and all the good folks at work who make your job a little easier. I could have gotten all pissed off thirty-something years ago when my wife Shirley tied my drunk ass to the bed with a clothesline and woke me up by beating me with a mop handle, but instead I figured I probably had it coming. Thinking back on it now, I realize I definitely had it coming. Instead of letting your thoughts think you into a corner, why not let them go? Letting go of your anger by simply exhaling it away makes room for the ultimate breath of fresh air. If someone's a jerk that's their misfortune, not yours.[65]

Well, there you have it. Just let it go. So simple when you say it like that, but for anyone over the age of three not so easy most of the time. Stress has a way of hanging on, especially when you live with a chronic challenge, and really, who doesn't? For me it is pain, but everyone I know could name at least one chronic stressor in his life at any given time. What I came to learn about stress during the time in my life that it hit me like a tsunami was this: stress builds on itself, and if you don't learn how to counteract the stress in your life with relaxation your body's go-to state will be stress. I experienced this during the year that my life resembled a bad country song. First my brother became deathly ill, then my relationship ended, my arthritis started

---

[65] Nelson, W., & Pipkin, T. (2006). The Willlie Way, Let it Go. In *The Tao of Willie: A guide to the happiness in your heart*. (p.68) New York: Gotham Books.

raging, and to top it all off my beloved dog died. My body entered into a tailspin and forgot how to be relaxed. Because of my long history of pain, this hyper-vigilant state was hard to stop. It took years of patient work with myself before I could sleep through the night without an herb or pill, and before I once again was able to experience feelings of joy inside without anxiety.

The reason why it takes such diligence to be calm and it is so easy to get riled up is because the stress circuit is so important for survival. Remember, if our ancestors hadn't been able to get into fight-or-flight mode at the drop of a hat we wouldn't be here today. Stress is easy to get into and not always so easy to get out of. That's why it is important to learn how to unravel stress in your life as soon as possible and to practice relaxation techniques daily. It can be as simple as taking a few deep breaths every so often and looking out the window at the trees. I've learned to become very good at recognizing when I'm feeling stressed, and when I do, to stop, figure out its source, and either do something about it or change my perspective so that once again I feel relaxed.

Life is full of things you have no choice about: pain, difficult circumstances, illness, and where and when you were born, to name just a few. These things can be extremely challenging and stressful. But you can choose not to add fuel to the fire. Keeping perspective, remaining aware of what's truly important, and staying in touch with the infinite wisdom of the universe through regularly connecting with the divine are ways that I've found to help me navigate the trials of life with grace. The keystone to self-care is learning how to move through stress with ease. Without a regular practice of stress management, you will forever remain stuck in disharmony and disease. And remember that you don't want to learn to swim when you are about to drown; a daily practice of relaxation will save the day when you really need it.

"Whenever you are sincerely pleased, you are nourished."
—Ralph Waldo Emerson[66]

Skepticism of pleasure permeates modern society. Get a massage and you run the risk of being viewed as a hedonist, but work an eighty-hour week and you'll rarely be accused of being a masochist. When I was twenty-seven, I decided to work part-

[66] Ralph Waldo Emerson. (n.d.). Retrieved from http://izquotes.com/quote/327915

time so that I could take care of my health. I knew that a forty-hour work week taxed my body too much and that I needed more time for sleep, rest, exercise, and yes, fun. Since then I've had countless people ask me in an incredulous tone, "How do you do it?" It's as if by working part-time I have one foot in the door of a life on the street. I reassure them that I'm just fine, thanks, and move the conversation to other things. I know that the extra money would be nice but my happiness is not dependent on it, and the joy I get from the extra free time I have is well worth it.

I have time for daily hikes, making my own food, seeing friends, resting, and meditation, and these things bring me great pleasure. I compare this to times in my life when I've been stuck in a grind of going through the motions of life with no time for fun, and it's as if I'm remembering a slow torture. I think that the reason why television is so popular is because most people are so exhausted at night it is the only form of entertainment they have energy for, the easiest way to pleasure. I've noticed that when I live in small Western U.S. towns fewer people have televisions and more people work part-time. They save money by harvesting fruit in the summer, getting out in the great outdoors, which costs only gas money, and driving used cars.

In the end, self-care is found in recognizing your needs and having the self-esteem to get them met. Make choices that come from a place of self-knowledge, empowerment, and authenticity, and you will find the ultimate expression of self-care, which is true love of self. Over time, your body will thank you, and begin to transform

LOVE

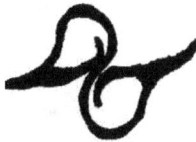

"*I have found the paradox, that if you love until it hurts there can be no more hurt, only love.*"

– Daphne Rae, Love Until it Hurts[67]

---

[67] Daphne Rae. (n.d.). Retrieved from http://www.goodreads.com/author/show/1989751.Daphne_Rae

Love is one of most misunderstood words in the English language. It can be said lightly, as in "I love cookies!" Dramatically: "I love him so much I can't live without him!" Universally: "Love makes the world go 'round!" One thing the word love never is, though: neutral. Love is all emotion; there is nothing rational about it. ("Love is blind.") We all crave love, it is a universal desire, and some would even argue, a necessity. Mother Theresa once said, "The hunger for love is much more difficult to remove than the hunger for bread." Love is seen in creatures great and small; it may just be the force that connects us all. Why then does it often seem so elusive?

Chandra Mohan Jain, otherwise known as Osho, was an Indian Mystic and professor of philosophy. He was no stranger to controversy; he famously criticized socialism, organized religion, Mahatma Ghandi, and advocated for a more open attitude towards sexuality. Osho spoke often and candidly about love. To Osho, love is experienced differently depending on how you choose to experience life. Osho said that there are as many loves as there are people; Adolph Hitler and Mahatma Ghandi will have extremely different ideas about what love is and will experience love very differently. Living in the many layers of love will be people who experience love in each layer. If you are living in a lower plane of existence, ruled by power, domination, and control, then that is how you will experience love. As you transcend this plane you will begin to experience love as a state of being, with no strings attached. Here is Osho:

> Everybody has their own idea of love. And only when you come to the state where all ideas about love have disappeared, where love is no more an idea but simply your being, then only will you know its freedom. Then love is God. Then love is the ultimate truth.[68]

Jesus Christ also embodied love. My favorite anecdotes from the Bible have always been the stories of Jesus washing the feet of lepers, who were the untouchables of his time. Foot washing was a common practice when visiting the home of another, but washing someone else's feet was only done by a slave. In choosing to wash the feet of people who were the pariahs in society, Jesus was committing a most humble and loving act. He endured the judgment and commentary about his actions with grace, and in doing so demonstrated what love is to us all.

[68] Osho (1931-1990) Motives-Love-Alchemical?- Osho Online Library. (n.d.). Retrieved from http%3A%2F%2Fwww.osho.com%2Fiosho%2Flibrary%2Fread-book%2Fonline-library-motives-love-alchemical-65b11a7f-823%3Fp%3Dc6cd4bb484605a2190977a1865c6fa6f

> Love is patient; love is kind; it does not envy, it does not boast, it is not proud. It is not rude, it is not arrogant or self-seeking. It is not easily angered, it keeps no records of wrongdoings, but rejoices in the truth. It does not insist on its own way; Love bears all things, believes all things, hopes all things, endures all things. Love never fails. (1 Corinthians 13:4-8a)

You can speak about love all day long, but true love can be seen. It is unconditional and without judgment. The actions of someone who understands what love is will look very different from someone who doesn't. Mother Teresa embodied this through her forty-nine years of service to the poor in Calcutta, India. Never interested in the attention her work garnered, when she received the Noble Peace Prize in 1979 she refused the traditional ceremonial banquet and asked that the $192,000 in funds used for the ceremony be given to the poor in India. When questioned about what people could do to promote world peace, she answered, "Go home and love your family."

> Love is a fruit in season at all times, and within reach of every hand. Anyone may gather it and no limit is set. Everyone can reach this love through meditation, spirit of prayer, and sacrifice, by an intense inner life.[69]

Don Miguel Ruiz is a bestselling author and a Nagual, or Shaman, in the Toltec tradition. He writes often and eloquently about love and the illusions we hold about ourselves and the world that keep us from being loving. Ancient Toltec wisdom tells us that everything we believe about ourselves and the world is a dream. From a very young age we are taught how to dream our dream by our family and society, and over time this dream becomes our reality. The collective dream is what creates life as we know it: rules, laws, religions, what is acceptable, desirable or not. Each of us go through our day hearing the thousands of voices that result from our collective dream, and, more often than not, we come up lacking. We are constantly comparing ourselves to a standard that has been created by our particular society, and from this standard we form our identity. Short, tall, thin, fat, smart, stupid, mean, nice, successful, loser, beautiful, ugly, sick, well; in the end all of these labels do nothing but harm because they are not based in love, but fear. "Do I measure up?" we ask ourselves when we

[69] Mother Teresa. (n.d.). Retrieved from http://en.wikiquote.org/wiki/Mother_Teresa

look in the mirror, and when we look at those around us. When we compare ourselves to others we are feeding the ego, by feeling better or less than. In our constant quest to keep up with the Jones, we forget that our name is Smith. We fail to recognize that we were made from love, and only in honoring our perfect uniqueness will we return to this love. Don Miguel Ruiz:

> Love coming out of you is the only way to be happy. Unconditional love for yourself. Complete surrender to that love for yourself. You no longer resist life. You no longer reject yourself. You no longer carry all that blame and guilt. You just accept who you are, and accept everyone else the way he or she is. You have the right to love, to smile, to share your love and to not be afraid to receive it also. That is the healing. Three simple points: the truth, forgiveness, and self-love. With these three points the whole world will heal and no longer be a mental hospital.[70]

To experience unfettered love one must look no further than a pet or small child. My dog Jasper reminds me every day how to love. His goofy nature and wagging tail don't change to spite me when I fail to take him on a hike. He doesn't question my intentions when I'm too tired to give him a good scratch. Jasper is always giving and receiving love even when his actions aren't appreciated. When Jasper was a puppy, I was dating a man who had little patience for him. He called Jasper incorrigible and said he was a bad dog. Everything Jasper did elicited a rolling of the eyes or a harsh word and sometimes even a swat. Jaspers' response to this treatment was to try harder and harder to demonstrate his love.

One particularly memorable example of this happened on one of the first camping trips we took together. We set up camp near a stream, and as soon as we got there Jasper proceeded to run straight for it. Not long after he came back, tail wagging, with a dead fish in his mouth. Robert's horrified look was enough to deflate Jasper, so he dropped it at Rob's feet. Rob immediately threw it into the trash. I sat back and watched what came next without comment. As soon as Rob turned his back little Jasper reached into the trash, took the fish out, walked into the tent and placed the fish on Rob's pillow. He sat there with a pleased-

---

[70] Ruiz, M. (1999). Healing the Emotional Body. In *The mastery of love: A practical guide to the art of relationship*. San Rafael, CA: Amber-Allen Pub.

as-punch look on his face. I stifled my laughs as well as I could and gently took the fish back to the stream it had come from. Over the years Rob was in his life Jasper never stopped trying, despite the fact that not once were his attempts at love appreciated.

How often do we treat our bodies the way Rob treated Jasper? Looking at it with disgust while reacting to its efforts to do the best it can by suppressing those efforts, silently calling it names. This body, the one we were born with and will die with, we tend to treat with disdain and lack of empathy. How many people do you know that love their body? How many people do you know who criticize their body at every opportunity? How many people do you know who are never satisfied with the pure attempts that their body makes to do the best it can? And then sabotage those attempts by not taking care of it? Our body is like a puppy. All it can do is love you back, try as hard as it can with the wisdom it was born with, and never give up. Unlike you, it won't judge. And yet, rarely does it get this level of care returned.

The dream that we collectively have created is set up for self-loathing. The images of models you see in magazines are not real people. They are air-brushed versions of people, yet we are supposed to look at them and think, "If only I bought that night cream I should be able to look like this." Cellulite doesn't exist in the media except in scandalous tabloids with headlines exclaiming, "Ms. J is getting FAT!!" Breasts are either too big or too small. Men aren't entirely immune to this either. There is always someone stronger, cooler, and more masculine to compare oneself to. Sadly, this self-loathing can start very young. As soon as a child enters school, they are tested to see how they compare with their peers. Reading, writing, arithmetic, and athletics: all of these activities are set up for competition and comparison. When did we lose the ability to be fine just the way we are?

I heard a story about the Dalai Lama once that I'll never forget. He was visiting the United States and giving a talk to a group of American Buddhist teachers. One of them raised a hand and asked, "How do you recommend we counsel our students who struggle with meditation and begin to feel that there is something wrong with them, that they are unworthy in some way?" The Dalai Lama had his interpreter repeat the question to him three times. The question flummoxed him; he couldn't

understand what they were asking. When he finally
understood, it took awhile for him to come up with an answer.
"In Tibet we grow up knowing that by being born we have
inherent worth. We never question this, because in our culture
we know that just by being born, we are born with a purpose
only we can fulfill. That purpose may include a grand life or a
simple one, but each has the same value. Feeling unworthy is
not possible because we are all inherently worthy; there is no
question. Please remind your students of this."

"To love oneself is the beginning of a lifelong romance."
–Oscar Wilde[71]

We all have a pattern of self-abuse. This pattern is learned from
family, society, and inherent traits. A person who is inherently
shy may worry more about what other people think of them. In
my case this self-abuse was one of denial and feeling unworthy.
Looking in the mirror I would only see the arthritis, and this
would isolate me in my mind. From a young age I told myself
that I was a leech on society, that because I had arthritis I had
nothing to offer. I couldn't do the things that other kids took for
granted and I needed so much extra time and attention. I
looked at those around me and saw normal; I looked at myself
and saw abnormal. In my mind, who would choose me when
they could have an upgraded version, one that didn't require so
much to keep it running? I would spend most of my energy
trying to prove to myself and others that this wasn't true. I kept
my happy mask on the majority of the time, allowing the
sadness and isolation to come out when my only company was
my dog Mandy. This pattern of stuffing negative feelings in,
never showing my anger and hopelessness to the world came to
a head when I was fourteen and developed anorexia.

When I stopped eating I had just started high school. All my
good friends were moving into varsity sports and dating. I was
never going to make any team at the varsity level, and I was
avoiding dating like the plague because I could only hide my
disease so well. Since I didn't talk about it a certain distance
was required, and dating would definitely be too close for
comfort. During this time I retreated into myself. I decided to do
the one thing I was good at and knew would garner a positive
reaction from my parents: stay thin. This decision was one that
would alter the course of my life. Staying small soon became

---

[71] Oscar Wilde. (n.d.). Retrieved from http://en.wikiquote.org/wiki/Oscar_Wilde

much more than a simple idea. It soon became my singular focus.

It eliminated the problems that puberty was threatening to bring. It also gave me the feeling of absolute power over a body that had done nothing but hurt me my entire conscious life. In my young mind I felt rejected by my body so I decided to reject it right back. I stopped feeding it, and I began to disappear. Before the anorexia came creeping in I never got angry, but this disease unleashed a fury of anger that surprised me. By rejecting myself, I was taking control of the only thing I had left: my willpower. The more I felt my life was careening out of my control, the more control I exerted over what I ate. I starved myself just enough to inflict great suffering on my already overwhelmed body, but not enough to kill it. This denial was done without any introspection or planning, yet in choosing anorexia I chose one of the most extreme ways to demonstrate the ultimate self-rejection. It was the opposite of self-love.

Once we begin to look at the ways we find ourselves wanting, we see this reflected in the way we live our life. Don Miguel Ruiz talks about how we choose partners that abuse and reject us in the way we abuse and reject ourselves. We tolerate this abuse up to a point, but if our partner crosses the line and inflicts more pain than we self-inflict, we leave. Over the years I have left men who began to cross the line from selfishness and lack of interest in my needs into cruelty, through an uncaring and disdainful attitude. I may have ignored my body's needs, and judged them harshly, but apart from the anorexia I'd never denied its basic needs. When my body was crying out for help, I'd show up. As I said, even when I had anorexia I fed it just enough to keep it alive. The men I chose would start out putting their needs above my own, ignoring my timid requests for extra rest or TLC and would eventually end up doing something that I couldn't in good faith make excuses for. After this it would take awhile, but I knew I'd have to leave.

A few years into my first long-term relationship, my boyfriend Derek began to change. He no longer asked about my pain level, stopped going to the doctor with me, and wasn't aware of what medication I was on anymore. One day I developed a paper cut at work. It didn't heal and it felt different, almost as if it wanted to muster up the energy required to do the job to patch my skin but it couldn't. At the time I was on a few immune suppressant drugs and it seemed like every other week I'd get an infection that required antibiotics. This time, I showed the cut to Derek. He shrugged and said, "Looks okay to me."

I had to agree but I knew that in this case looks were deceiving. Sure enough, that Monday I woke up with red streaks moving down my arm. I knew enough to go to the hospital where I received a diagnosis of cellulitis and was put on IV antibiotics. The doctor told me, "You can either stay in the hospital for five days, or you can go home with the IV needle in your arm and come back every day for treatment." Of course I chose to go home, which in retrospect may not have been the best choice. All week Derek made food without an offer to make some for me, let dishes pile in the sink, invited his friends over to the tiny house where we were living who inevitably glanced my way and asked, "What's wrong with your arm?" I was used to sucking it up and not complaining, but really, if there ever was a time to demonstrate caring this was it. During that week I imagined life with Derek 2, 3, 10 years down the road and it wasn't an appealing vision. A few months later we said goodbye.

This theme with the men I chose to bring into my life would be repeated, time and again, throughout my twenties and thirties. Deep down I felt unworthy because of my self-perceived damaged body, so I dated people who were self-concerned, uncurious about who I really was, and more interested in a temporary playmate than a long-term partner. I would spend days pushing myself at whatever activity they enjoyed and then go home to recover alone. I would get the sleep I needed, eat the food that my body liked, and once I was rested up I'd go back for more fun. Over the years I learned to rock climb, ride horses, ski moguls, mountain bike, shoot a gun (happily for everybody I only had to do this once, and when I literally hit the side of a barn the gun was taken away from me), and drive huge trucks around an Australian property. I told myself how much fun I was having learning new things, and I really did have fun. The actual activities I was enjoying weren't the problem. The problem was that I was so gung ho because it helped me to hide, to prove to myself and my boyfriends that I was "normal," and "acceptable." During my twenties I would inevitably start dating someone in the spring when my body felt better and the relationship would end in the winter when I needed more rest. Usually it was a mutual decision; I had stopped being so available for fun and they were beginning to wear me out with their blissfully ignorant, self-involved attitude. This pattern fed into my need to be accepted and also, ironically, proved to me just how unworthy I was. I was reflecting the pattern of my self-abuse back to myself through my relationships.

I finally understood this when I had an ah-ha moment a few years ago. I was watching the movie, *Runaway Bride*, and realized that Julia Roberts' character and I had a lot in common. In the movie she got engaged to men and then ran away on the day of the wedding as she was walking up the altar. Richard Gere plays a reporter who comes to town to do a story on her, a few weeks before her fourth attempt at marriage. During the time they spend together her tells her, "You weren't being supportive, you were scared. You are the most lost woman I know. You are so lost you don't even know what kind of eggs you like!" Apparently, with each fiancé she ate a different kind of eggs, poached, scrambled, egg whites only, and each man was convinced that this was her favorite. She was hiding behind a carefree, happy façade because she was afraid to step into her own authentic shoes. Like Julia's character, I had become a chameleon, creating a façade with each man I was with so I didn't have to face the reality of who I was.

My version of self-abuse was extreme and took years to soften. The pattern of abuse was set up subconsciously, and unwound consciously. This unwinding is a lifelong process that requires daily practice and much patience. It began when I got tired of acting out against myself. I had to admit that even though my body was unruly and hurt me I actually had very tender feelings towards it. I looked at the things I did to torture myself, including harsh judgments I made, not feeding it enough, and pretending it was unattractive. Then began to look at the things I did to protect it.

What I've found is that even though we may be trained from a young age to criticize and reject ourselves, this isn't really our natural state. When given the opportunity, we all can learn to shine. Deep down there is a star within us all, and to be healthy one must do the work to let the star shine through. As I've said before, you must be your own best friend. After all, you will be living with yourself for the rest of your life. Why would you want to live with a critical, judgmental self when you can have a loving, caring, compassionate one?

When I actually looked at myself with an undistorted mirror, I found plenty of things to be proud of and to love. My strong willpower, my endurance, my curiosity, my never-give-up attitude, my optimism, and a body that despite great pain did amazing things and was more active than most. When I stopped comparing myself to others I began to see more clearly and realized for the first time just how special, and even desirable, I was. I began to be truly kind to myself and was surprised at how easy this was. If someone like me, who has gone to extremes of self-abuse and self-denial for most of my life can turn my inner life into one of kindness, anyone can.

"The sun never says to the earth,
"You owe me."
Look what happens with a love like that.
It lights up the whole sky."
–Hafiz[72]

Many people talk about the power of forgiveness. One of my favorite mentors is Caroline Myss, an author and medical intuitive. She talks often about forgiveness, saying that forgiveness is a necessity for healing. The inability to forgive yourself or others will end up draining your energy, your power, and your emotional resources. According to Caroline, the inability to forgive is the strongest poison to the human spirit. Forgiveness is one of the richest gifts you can give yourself. It will transform your life and your thoughts. Once you learn to forgive you free up an immense amount of emotional energy that can be used to heal yourself and your life. I've found this to be true. In my case, the person I most had to forgive was myself. I had to forgive myself for almost taking my own life, for abusing my struggling body, for denying my body the rest and care that it desperately needed, for hiding my true self from others, and for berating it whether it was feeling good or bad.

For me, forgiveness is the nectar that has fed my journey to health. It seeps into the hopelessness and transforms it. It brings me out from under the weight I've carried and shows me that I am worthy of love. Forgiveness whispers sweet words into my starving soul and reflects back to me what I've always hoped for, but never believed. Forgiveness has transformed me; it has brought me to a place where I can love myself and reflect this love to all those around me. Forgiveness takes practice,

---

[72] Piper, R. (2013, May 01). 10 Life-Changing Lessons Inspired By Hafiz. Retrieved May 1, 2013, from http://www.mindbodygreen.com/0-8883/10-life-changing-lessons-inspired-by-hafiz.html

and like most worthwhile endeavors, patience. After a lifetime of playing the blame game you can't just flip a switch into loving kindness. Once you realize how important forgiveness is you have to learn to close the door on blame and walk toward a life where your compassion over-rides your need to assign fault. When you practice sending love out to those who have hurt you, or the things you've done to hurt yourself, you begin to remember that inside the deep hurt you've felt there is always a lesson. Learning the lesson contained within the hurt makes you stronger, wiser, and more humane. It helps you to understand what love really is.

The opposite to love, despite what many people think, isn't hate. It is apathy. Witnessing apathy is the saddest and most unforgettable experience, one that sears its image into your soul. When I think of apathy I picture caged animals in zoos, factory farms, or medical testing facilities. The look in their eyes says it all; it is beyond betrayal, beyond despair, beyond pain. I also think of some of the patients I've had when I've worked in nursing homes, who shrivel inside themselves when you enter the room and refuse to acknowledge your presence. These people are our untouchables, forgotten by their families and waiting to die. They usually get their wish sooner rather than later. Love for them is a distant memory, a faint wispy thread that they can no longer grasp.

Apathy was described by Victor Frankl in his memoir *Man's Search For Meaning*, about his experiences as a prisoner during the holocaust. Apathy for Frankl was a sure way to put one foot in the grave. The word apathy comes from the Greek, meaning without feeling. A life with no feeling will eliminate any chance to imbue love, the feeling that permeates everything. As Victor Hugo once said, "It's nothing to die; it's frightful not to live."[73] Where does apathy come from? How does it take root in the human soul? This is a question for great thinkers, but also one that we all need to ask because it is one thing that will kill any hope for healing.

During my years working in nursing homes I was able to see apathy up close almost every day, and as a therapist it was my worst fear. Give me a cantankerous old man any day, the kind that would hurl obscenities at you when you walked through his door. I knew that this superficial anger and hate was masking

[73] "Les Misérables/Volume 5/Book Ninth/Chapter 5." Les Miserables/Volume 5/ Book Ninth/Chapter 5. Wikisource, the Free Online Library, n.d. Web. 29 May 2015.

fear of un-love, fear that he wasn't being cared for or about. This verbal (and sometimes physical) firestorm could be transformed with kind acts and validation. I knew that someone who cared enough to yell at me still had it in him to fight for his life.

Apathy begins alongside hopelessness, purposelessness, lack of control and, as Frankl described, witnessing or being a part of horrific experiences such as those seen in war. Once apathy sets in there is nothing left to live for. One of my most unforgettable patients was the first client I ever saw during my time working at the Salt Lake City, Utah, Veterans Hospital. He had been referred to me so that I could evaluate him for adaptive equipment that would allow him to be safer in his home. He was in his eighties, a tiny, frail man that made even me, a person that only breaks three digits on the scale on a good day, look like Goliath. I began to talk to him about his home life and he mentioned that he had difficulty sleeping. "How long has this been going on?" I inquired. "Sixty-five years. For sixty-five years I've had the same nightmare. I wake up in the night striking out and my wife has to wake me. For a few years we've been tying a rope around my ankle and she tugs on it when I start thrashing because she's not strong enough anymore to wake me up any other way."

After I had picked my jaw up from the floor I asked him if he remembered his dreams. "Sure I do, it's been the same all this time. I dream about the people I killed in World War II." He then proceeded to tell me that he had been a sniper in the Philippines. He was helicoptered into remote areas and left for days where he was instructed to shoot any enemy soldiers that he saw. He was very good at what he did; he would see a rustle in a branch 1000 yards away and shoot at it. The rustle would stop. Occasionally, though, it didn't and he knew that the man he had just shot was still alive. With nothing to do but think, he would picture his target bleeding and dying slowly. This thought would torture him until he couldn't take it anymore. Then he would move over to the spot where the injured man was lying and put a bullet in his brain. This eighteen-year-old kid had become a killer, and for the next sixty-five years he would torture himself because of it.

My patient then asked me a question: "Am I going to hell?" I took a few seconds to consider my answer. "No," I said. "You aren't going to hell. You've been suffering for sixty-five years now, God won't want you to suffer any more than you already

have." His eyes teared up, and I could see him change in front of
me. His shoulders moved back, and his breath became deeper.
It was as if he was allowing himself to breathe in life for the first
time since the war. He left my office and I never saw him after
that day, but I'd like to think that this little man began to love
himself again, even just a little bit, at the age of eighty-five.
As Victor Frankl describes in the following passage, the
antidote to apathy is love:

> A thought transfixed me: for the first time in my life I
> saw the truth as it is set into song by so many poets,
> proclaimed as the final wisdom by so many thinkers.
> The truth — that love is the ultimate and the highest
> goal to which man can aspire. Then I grasped the
> meaning of the greatest secret that human poetry and
> human thought and belief have to impart: The salvation
> of man is through love and in love.[74]

Ultimately, apathy and love are a choice we all can make. We
decide whether we want to live in love, or in apathy. It doesn't
matter what you've done in the past. You have the opportunity
every minute of every day to choose differently, and there is so
much to be gained by choosing to love and be loved.

Love and Be Loved. This is a mantra that I say to myself every
day. It reminds me of my truth, the truth that I choose to honor
on behalf of myself and others. Like most things that are
worthwhile in life it takes effort, especially the love of self, but
for me, there is no other choice. Osho says that we don't need to
learn how to love, we need to unlearn un-love. Love is our
natural state; un-love we learn, and unfortunately throughout
our lives there are plenty of opportunities to learn un-love.
When the society in which we find ourselves encourages
competition, fear, self-loathing and divisiveness, love becomes
harder to believe in. When most of the love relationships we see
revolve around possession our view of love can easily become
skewed.

"Your task is not to seek for love, but merely to seek and find all
the barriers within yourself that you have built against it."
-Rumi[75]

[74] Frankl, V. (1957). *Mans Search For Meaning*. Pg 57 New York, NY: Pocket Books.
[75] Crystal, D. (n.d.). BBC World Service/ Learning English/Moving Words. Retrieved from
http://www.bbc.co.uk/worldservice/learningenglish/movingwords/quotefeature/rumi.shtml

Unlearning un-love has to happen before true love can grow in your heart. It involves recognizing where un-love exists in your inner and outer worlds, and then choosing to become love instead. Sounds easy, right? You are a very loving person, correct? Okay then, look in the mirror and see where your thoughts go. How many criticisms do you hatch up for yourself? You've already slipped into un-love. Turn on the television and watch any reality show. Is there any love there at all? Or are you seeing competition, gossip, and mean-spirited pettiness? Let's keep moving outward into our greater society. How about, ahem, politics? Is there anything patient, kind, forgiving, truthful, non-boastful, non-self-seeking, or non-judgmental about politics? Okay, let's look at our relationship to those around the globe. Our country is a melting pot, right? Doesn't the Statue of Liberty say, "Give me your tired, your poor, your huddled masses yearning to breathe free; the wretched refuse of your teeming shore, send these, the homeless, tempest-tossed to me!" I guess she never got the memo about the huge fence we are building down South to keep out those pesky South Americans.

Now, let's go back to the personal. How truly loving are your relationships? This is a time for honesty. With your intimate partner, are you forgiving when they don't live up to your expectations? Are you jealous when they appear to outperform you? Are you more concerned about what you are getting than what you are giving? Truly loving someone means that you wake up every day and resolve to love you partner more, without any expectation of receiving anything in return. Do you understand that in a loving relationship each person is responsible for their own happiness? No one else makes you happy; they can only influence your experience. Can you love and respect yourself enough to leave a relationship that no longer serves you? When you really examine your life, you begin to realize that truly loving is the easiest and hardest thing you'll ever do.

Loving starts with the self. Sometimes I wish everyone could just hit a reboot button in their bodies and forget all the things they've decided to hate about themselves. If we could all just focus on being happy just as we are it would be natural to allow our true beauty to shine through. Life would still continue to challenge us, but our reactions would be entirely different. Many of us would choose different jobs, friends, and partners.

Self-love really is the way to a wholly satisfying, rich and healthy life. It is the only way one can begin to love others. Love is the greatest gift one can give, the sweetest state of being one can experience, the most unconditional act one can perform, and the salvation of us all.

CONNECTION

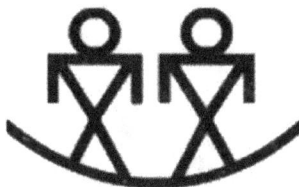

"The best thing to hold onto in life is each other."
–Audrey Hepburn[77]

---

[76] "Brothers Symbol." *Brothers Symbol*. N.p., n.d. Web. 01 June 2015.
[77] Audrey Hepburn quote. (n.d.). Retrieved from
http://www.brainyquote.com/quotes/quotes/a/audreyhepb378280.html

The road to true health, despite its many un-sharable moments, is not one to be walked alone. Sadly, the modern experience of chronic illness encourages separateness. Medical doctors will only listen to complaints about the specific symptoms they are trained to handle, and appear uninterested in any organ that isn't relevant for them. The emotional aspects of disease are rarely addressed by medical doctors, and if they are, usually take the form of a referral to counseling or a prescription for a pill. Families are left to figure it out as they go, and individuals with disease are unsure about when to disclose anything to their employer for fear of discrimination. Not wanting to be a burden, most people try to suck it up and navigate the immense task of managing their illness with as little assistance as possible from others. Often, even partners are kept in the dark for fear that they will begin to feel like a caregiver. When did disease become such a lonely experience?

Native cultures have an extremely different worldview of health and disease. The National Aboriginal Health Strategy says this about Aboriginal views on health:

> "Health" to Aboriginal peoples is a matter of determining all aspects of their life, including control over their physical environment, of their dignity, of community self-esteem, and of justice. It is not merely a matter of the provision of doctors, hospitals, medicine or the absence of disease and incapacity. ... Health is not just the physical well-being of an individual but the social, emotional and cultural well being of the whole community. This is a whole-of-life view and includes the cyclical concept of life-death-life. **Even if only one person is sick, the whole community hurts.**[78]

There lies the crux of the difference between a Native worldview and that of modern culture. In Native cultures healing is greater than the self. The community knows that the health of each person is vital for the health of the whole. This means that in Native societies, healing is a group effort that includes ceremonies, dancing, prayers, and chanting. Healing involves trust that the ill person will never be abandoned; they are able to lay down the load of illness at the feet of others who will join them on their quest for health.

---

[78] BULLINAH AHS. (n.d.). Retrieved from http://www.bullinahahs.org.au/about-us/aboriginal-definition-of-health/

Contrast this to the modern approach of isolating the sick, offering rational advice and sympathy while true connection with the ill is the exception rather than the rule. Modern culture has become so enamored with reductionism, or reducing complex systems into simpler systems, it has forgotten that parts are always connected to the whole whether you are talking about parts of the body, parts of the environment, or individuals in a community. The innate curiosity about how things work which drives the scientific method encourages tunnel vision and people end up seeing the trees without the forest. With all the resources modern technology can provide this basic fact remains: healing doesn't happen by looking through a microscope, in a sterile hospital room, or a lab. It happens through connection. Without a healthy connection to our inner and outer environment we will never be healthy.

The medical traditions of First Nations Peoples and Native Americans in North America, as well as the traditional Eastern medical model, understand illness and health in the context of balance. Balance in all things: spiritual, mental, and physical, and harmony with the community and environment creates health. Imbalance in any of these areas can contribute to disease. This is reflected in the Medicine Wheel, which has been used for many centuries by indigenous cultures such as the Native Americans in the Northern United States and Southern Canada. A medicine wheel symbolizes the circle of life and includes the directions North, South, East, and West. Each direction has a color, element (fire, earth, air, water), a season (Winter, Spring, Summer, Fall), and characteristics (wisdom, intuition, manifestation, trust, creation, intellect). The center of the wheel is creation, representing balance and harmony. The medicine wheel is used to heal disease by focusing on where balance has been lost, and in doing so, unearthing the cause of the illness. Just looking at a medicine wheel, one can imagine how using one for healing might result in a drastic shift in how one views one's self and the world.

The use of the medicine wheel is unique to each community and is based on oral traditions that are kept sacred. In representing the cycles of life, the wheel represents the holistic way that Native cultures see their world. Throughout life everyone passes through a series of cycles; these cycles are connected to all other living things, the earth and spirit. By seeing life in this way, it becomes clear how related each of our actions are to each other and to the environment in which we live. By stepping into the wheel, one begins to understand how to be a better person, to find the individual right path through truth, knowledge, connection, and wisdom. Without this, healing cannot happen.

"A healthy social life is found only, when in the mirror of each soul the whole community finds its reflection, and when in the whole community the virtue of each one is living."
–Rudolf Steiner[79]

The founding fathers knew how crucial interdependence woven throughout daily life is, and that a healthy community isn't possible without healthy individuals. They crafted many of the key ideas in the Constitution after consulting and being influenced by the Iroquois Nation, and Iroquois chiefs were invited to the Constitutional Congress. Sadly, as modern society has grown up it has grown away from its roots. We've forgotten that if we poison our soil we poison ourselves, that if we isolate ourselves in a huge Mc Mansion the people around us will never be able to reach out when we are in need, that by focusing so much on material wealth we fail to remember that true wealth is when a body is free from disease and fully loved. By not respecting the unseen forces of nature and the human spirit, our ego may be inflated but our healthy balance is forever lost.

His Holiness, the 14th Dalai Lama, was once interviewed by a young man who had spent time in Palestine reporting on the seemingly never-ending conflict there. He asked the Dalai Lama his opinion on how to finally achieve peace in the Middle East. He answered, "I think the first step is to cool negative emotions, more festivals, more picnics, let them forget about these emotions, make a personal friend, then talk about serious matters." It is easy to forget about the healing power of coming together, spending time with others when there is nothing on the agenda but having fun. The healthiest families, partnerships, workplaces, and societies are ones in which laughter often fills the air. Who knows, maybe sometimes healing is as simple as a festival.

This reminds me of a story I read about Ghengis Khan. I know, he was a bloodthirsty savage; what did he know about peace or community? Actually, a lot. It always amazes me to think about

---

[79] Rudolf Steiner. (n.d.). Retrieved from http://izquotes.com/quote/177486

how one man, born on the desolate steppes of Mongolia, to a
family who was tossed out of society and left to die because his
father had been killed, managed to transform the entire world
in many positive ways. Mongol law prohibited blood feuds,
adultery, theft, and bearing false witness. Trade routes were
opened up forever after throughout Europe and Asia, and art
and culture blossomed for hundreds of years in countries such
as Iran under the influence of these routes. But the thing that
makes me smile the most when I think of Ghengis Khan is how
curious and non-judgmental he was about religion.
Throughout his life he changed religions according to which
religion fascinated him, and he consulted often with religious
scholars. In his home city he constructed a town square that
had buildings from every religion next to each other. The
mosque was next to the temple, which was next to the church.
People who wanted to worship had to walk to the same place
and I imagine they talked and visited before and after they
worshipped. Ghengis Khan's insatiable curiosity about religion
led him to have a festival. During this festival there was a
debate among the religious leaders from each major religious
tradition. The rules were as follows: A question would be posed
and each cleric would answer in turn without interruption.
Voices were not to be raised, fighting was not allowed, and after
each question everyone had to take a drink of fermented milk.
You can imagine how much fun the debate became after the
first five questions. Ghengis Khan may have been savage, but
he knew a thing or two about how to bring people together.
When you share space with others you eventually have to get
along.

Years ago I worked as an occupational therapist in a locked
Alzheimer's care facility. The people living there had at one
time been captains of industry, doctors, and teachers. Even one
of the original animators for the Walt Disney company came
through the door at one point. Before disease took away their
ability to form complex thought, every single one of our
residents had a very high IQ. Day after day, I'd walk in and
wonder why. Why had this happened to such bright people,
people who had so much to offer with their brainpower? Why
did a disease like Alzheimer's, which destroys a person's brain,
personality, and uniqueness until they become a shell of their
former selves even exist?

What I saw as I walked through the hallways were physical
bodies whose souls had already left them. I would teach these
people how to continue to brush their teeth, encouraging rote

movements that would bring back muscle memory. I would watch as they paced the hallways and would tell them, "Your Mom is coming here soon to pick you up," when they became anxious about getting to school. The people who could still talk were usually living in a different time, sometimes convinced that they were ten years old. Whenever they would pass a mirror I would see a horrified look of disbelief as they tried to work out what this old person was doing staring back at them.

Dark humor permeated the facility among the employees. What is the best thing about having Alzheimer's? Getting to wake up every day with a different woman. It helped keep us from crying as we saw our beloved patients lose the ability to eat. With each of my patients I would enter a different time period. I would engage in conversations that would leave me shaking my head and continuing to ask why. Isn't life hard enough? Why does anyone need to be stripped of his personhood at the end? What kind of cruel cosmic joke was going on? I was not appreciating God's sense of humor.

These questions came to a head when there was an incident in the nursing home. As things go in the workplace, facts fluttered around in hushed whispers and became the telephone game as the facts were removed and insinuation grew. What I heard was that one of our cute little female residents cut another one with a pair of scissors. The cuts were along the inner thigh and near the vagina. Immediately, worst-case scenarios came to mind. Finally the Alzheimer's had turned someone violent. Maybe Doris imagined that Jean was having an affair with her husband, and she was exacting revenge. This would not be too big of a stretch; there were many affairs going on in the facility; usually these affairs took the form of two ancient people sharing kisses, hugs, and beds. When this happened the wives and husbands would be informed, everyone fully aware that the "cheaters" had no idea they were cheating because they didn't remember being married. Usually the spouses would let them carry on, wishing only happiness and comfort for their husband or wife in their final days. Because most of the residents were living in the past, occasionally someone would revisit a trauma that they had never emotionally dealt with. Every time I witnessed this it would happen to a woman who had been raped and never talked about it. This trauma would re-emerge as she began to talk about a man in her bedroom doing bad things, or hiding under the bed until nighttime when they would come out to ravage her. So, the thought that perhaps Doris had been cheated on and was acting out some long-held fantasy was in the realm of possibility.

As my imagination was contemplating this new terrible reality, another cruel aspect to this evil disease, I finally talked to someone who knew the facts. Little Doris, who weighed seventy-five pounds soaking wet on a good day, thought Jean was in trouble and was cutting off her clothes so she could save her. It turned out that Doris was re-enacting an old memory, the memory of when she was a nurse in WWII and performed triage. She was doing everything she could to help.

Jean was perfectly fine. The offending pair of scissors was locked away as they should have been to begin with, and life went on. For some reason, though, as I left for the day I couldn't stop crying. I felt as if an elephant had stepped on my chest. Luckily, it was a Friday and I had the weekend off. I spent the weekend both trying to understand my reaction to this event and attempting to find answers to the questions that plagued me.

It took some time, but what I finally came to understand changed my life. I had my own trauma that I hadn't fully dealt with. This disease was personal for me; my grandmother died of Alzheimer's, and although she was alive until I was twenty, I never really knew her. The woman I knew tried to put the iced cake in the oven. She ran away from her home and husband every day, convinced she was a young girl and this old man in the house had kidnapped her. She would say the wrong words for things, called apples peaches, and I would giggle. I never knew the amazing women who had traveled around Europe when she was young, who married a man that adored her, the math teacher who kept a beautiful home and baked the most amazing pies, the stellar bridge player. Although I'd never admitted it to myself, I felt robbed, cheated, and angry at my Grandma's fate. Working every day with people who reminded me of her was slowly rubbing salt into my long-held wound.

As I raged against the reality of a world that included Alzheimer's I began to play devil's advocate. What if there was a gift hidden inside the chaos of this disease? What would that gift be? I immediately came up with many. People with Alzheimer's teach the rest of us many, many lessons. Patience, kindness, the ability to see that we all live in our own dream, gratitude, the ability to love when our love can't be returned in the ways that are familiar. Maybe people with Alzheimer's are all giving us the selfless gift of teaching us how to be better people. From then on, my job and my world changed.

"We all take different paths in life, but no matter where we go we take a little of each other with us." –Tim McGraw[80]

I began to realize that even those people in the most dire of situations, who at first glance are completely dependent on others, are able to give. The gifts we receive from others are not always comfortable, especially when they come in the form of mirrors. I always prided myself on my patience until I had to stand in the room of a person with Alzheimer's for an hour and a half while I aided them in dressing independently. My self-assessed grip on reality was secure until I recognized the ease with which I entered the alternate realities of my patients. I began to see that there is no such thing as a complete dependent. Each of us, by sharing our lives with each other, is teaching, learning, loving, and growing. The men and women who have completely lost their mental abilities continue to teach those around them by providing a mirror. They remind everyone just how tenuously we all hold onto our "superior, evolved" brainpower. They reflect back to us our limits of patience; they bring stark light to how easily we are embarrassed. This tragic disease, by showing us a reflection of ourselves, keeps us humble.

Many years later I received a query from an associate who has a relationship website. He asked if I would write an article for him. "Can you write an advice column for spouses who are caregivers of people with rheumatoid arthritis?" A few days earlier I had fielded a question when being interviewed for a radio program. The interviewer asked me, "Has your Mom always been your primary caregiver?" Without waiting for an answer he went on, "How has she handled the ups and downs of your disease?" I had to stop for a few seconds; there were two different questions there. The very thought of me needing a caregiver, ever, had never crossed my mind. "Well, my Mom and I haven't lived in the same state since I was sixteen but when I was young she was definitely the one who took care of me on a day-to-day basis. It is hard for her to see me in pain and to know what she can do to help me ease it." I began to wonder if caregiving was the new buzzword in health-care. The more I

[80] Tim McGraw Quotes. (n.d.). Retrieved from
http://www.goodreads.com/author/quotes/35730.Tim_McGraw

thought about it the more it bothered me. I decided not to write about being a caregiver for a spouse with arthritis; instead I wrote an article on how to cope with living with rheumatoid arthritis vicariously.

The truth was my Mom and I had never really talked about how she handled living with my disease. There is a learning curve for anyone living with someone who has a disease. When it isn't your body it can be hard to understand, especially when your loved one lives with chronic pain. For me this was a worthwhile topic to explore. However, introducing the idea that one spouse will be a caregiver is dangerous. Once you enter the realm of caregiver and dependent you encourage burnout and passivity. You will be focused on your duties or your dependency and forget that every relationship is always a two-way street. You will begin to only see the disease and can become blind to the health and wisdom that lies beneath. The idea that one person in a relationship has to be the caregiver will inevitably make the person being cared for feel less than worthy and the caregiver feel trapped, perpetually exhausted or feeling guilty because they are taking time for themselves.

The worst thing about the idea of caregiving is that it fosters separateness. Instead of bringing two people together it divides them, which encourages isolation. It creates a child and a sitter, instead of two adults managing a challenge together. I've seen this in plenty of my patients. They come into the therapy room with their spouse and defer to them, talk less, and appear much more disabled than when I see them alone. They confide in me that their spouse has stopped asking for sex. They tell me that they feel insignificant and worthless. Their spouse always looks tired and acts as if the depth of their love is being tested every day.

In any long-term relationship there will be times when one person is incapacitated and needs a lot of help. In order to manage a sustained need in a healthy way two things have to happen. Support from the community has to come in and the flow of care has to remain open both ways. The healthiest couple I ever met dealt with a chronic disease called myasthenia gravis. This disease causes severe progressive muscle weakness. It can make it difficult to eat, walk, see, breathe, and even hold your head up. Bonnie had dealt with this disease for many years by the time I met her and her husband Mark. They were in their 50s; Mark worked, and although

Bonnie couldn't work anymore every day she did what she could to keep the house clean and meals made. Sometimes Bonnie couldn't do anything but relax and rest, and on those days she spent her time reading. They were obviously very much in love and spoke frankly about how the myasthenia gravis had changed their lives.

What I noticed as I heard them talk was that Mark highly respected his wife for facing severe weakness like a gladiator faced his enemy; she was fearless. She loved to garden and even though her garden was tiny it was immaculate. She never stopped being very much his wife, doing nice, thoughtful things for him whenever she had the energy. They shared a strong religious belief, had much in common, and always had lots to talk about. Neither Mark nor Bonnie held back in talking to each other or to me about how nasty her disease was. Sometimes they would be at a restaurant and suddenly she would realize that her muscles were too weak to swallow. Later they'd tell me about it, laughing together about how she managed to discreetly spit out her food into a napkin without anyone seeing.

Mark and Bonnie could easily have fallen into the caregiver/dependent cycle, but it never occurred to them. They both understood that despite her physical limitations, Bonnie never stopped being a kind, beautiful, intelligent, compassionate person, and still very much a woman. She never stopped making an effort to look nice in front of her husband. Mark knew this and it made him admire her even more. They hugged and kissed each other; even the touching they did when Mark had to help her was affectionate. And they never hesitated to call on their family and friends when they both needed a hand. Sometimes Mark wanted to go hunting, and their son would spend the weekend with Bonnie. They would pack in quality time and laugh a lot. The family was intact and healthy, and even when they cried, they cried together.

"Two are better than one, If one falls down, his friend can help him up. But pity the man who falls and has no one to help him up! Though one may be overpowered, two can defend themselves. A cord of three strands is not quickly broken."
–King Solomon Ecclesiastes 4:9-12
New International Version (NIV)

The first day of graduate school I stepped into the elevator of my new dorm. I had just arrived in New York City and was getting used to the constant noise. Even eleven stories above the street it seemed like I could hear sirens every twenty minutes. A bit apprehensive about what I was getting myself into with occupational therapy school and trying to appear well-rested, I was surprised to hear a voice call out from the corner of the elevator, "Hi there! What program are you in?" I turned to see a friendly face that belonged to my new lifelong friend, Kiki. It turned out that of all the thousands of students I could have met in the elevator, it was a kindred spirit that showed up. From that moment on Kiki and I were inseparable. One of the many reasons Kiki and I were two peas in a pod was that we both shared the all-too-real ability to walk in the shoes of our patients. I had a physical issue, juvenile rheumatoid arthritis, and she had dyslexia.

Two years later we decided to do our school internships together in Colorado. We arrived at our first internship, an inpatient ward for people with mental illnesses of all kinds. It's funny what daunts a person. Here we were, in a locked unit surrounded by people so ill that they thought they were Jesus Christ, a man who had pled insanity after murdering his daughter's boyfriend and a supervisor who barely showed up to check in on us; I was nervous about the fact that I couldn't open the paint jars during afternoon therapeutic craft groups. Kiki, on the other hand, was afraid that someone would catch on to her horrible spelling. So we did what best friends do; she loosened all the paint jars at the beginning of group for me and I re-read her notes, correcting all her spelling mistakes. It was a win-win situation that turned our insecurities into a private joke that lightened our load and brought us closer together.

Asking for support, despite how big your need appears to you in your head, is no big deal when it comes down to it. There is always something you can offer in return even if it is just a smile and a heartfelt thanks. Down the road you will pay it forward.

One brutal truth about living with chronic disease is that it constantly reminds you of just how alone each of us is in our experience. The immense task of living with disease isn't something anyone can ever fully share because most of disease has to be experienced to understand. Honestly, there are many things one would prefer not to share. The physical scars of disease don't compare to the daily hits to a person's self-esteem. The loss of many qualities you once took for granted can be wiped out in one fell swoop, and what is left is often someone you don't recognize. When this happens the people around you will begin to treat you differently and you will wonder who, exactly, they are seeing when they look at you. In my own experience, I've sometimes felt like an animal in a cage as I listen to those around me talk about me as if I weren't there, commenting on my limp or my stoic attitude, or some other aspect of myself that had shown up unbidden in a reaction to constant pain. I've also noticed how my efforts at connecting with others throughout my life has changed along with the inner changes that I've been so steadfast in creating.

When I was younger, I would isolate myself from others when the pain was too bad to hide; this isolation only served to make me feel worse about myself and my life. I desperately wanted someone who would be with me in my experience, without imposing their own fear and need onto me. Later, with the insight that years of observation and reflection can bring, I realized that this is why so many people with chronic illness become depressed. As an occupational therapist, I routinely saw people who stopped trying to connect to others because their attempts would only result in them feeling more isolated as they listened to unsolicited advice, sympathetic yet condescending words, or other people's fear about their situation. After being subjected to this enough times it is understandable that one will shut down, stop trying, and give up on the hope for any true connection, resigning one's self to a life alone.

The challenge is to cultivate companionship even when you are feeling at your lowest, because this is when you need it the most. It is a courageous act to keep trying to connect with others when you are feeling completely alone.

"Everyone hears what you say. Friends listen to what you say. Best friends listen to what you don't say." –Unknown[81]

Parker J. Palmer, writer, teacher, activist, and founder of the Center for Courage and Renewal, wrote these words in his book *Let Your Life Speak: Listening for the Voice of Vocation*:

---

[81] 43 Most Insightful Friendship Quotes. (n.d.). Retrieved from
http://www.lifeoptimizer.org/2007/10/10/43-most-insightful-friendship-quotes/

My evidence comes in part from my journey through clinical depression, from the healing I experienced as a few people found ways to be present me without violating my soul's integrity. Because they were not driven by their own fears, the fears that lead us either to "fix or abandon each other, they provided me with a lifeline to the human race. That lifeline constituted the most profound form of leadership I can imagine—leading a suffering person back to life from a living death. [82]

In his book he talks about being in the midst of depression. During this time he would sit alone for days in his house unable to function. One of his friends would come to his house, sit with him and massage his feet. There was no commentary about the state he was in or what he needed to do, just pure companionship. The very act of sitting with him, not turning away because the view wasn't pretty, and respecting his solitary journey, helped Parker to come back from his abyss. He goes on to say:

> The key to this form of community involves holding a paradox—the paradox of having relationships in which we protect each other's aloneness. We must come together in ways that respect the solitude of the soul, that avoid the unconscious violence we do when we try to save each other, that evoke our capacity to hold another life in ways that honor its mystery, never trying to coerce the other into meeting our own needs. [83]

Therein lies the key to true companionship: the ability to just be with the other person, to be a witness to their experience, to share in their joy and pain, unwavering and loving in your devotion to his life. It is the ability to accept life on life's terms for yourself and for each other. With time and as I grew wiser about my needs and the dangers of isolation, I have been able to find my own people who will simply be with me and let me be with them as we travel through life together.

Here is another paradox: there is no need to fix anything in another's life, especially when it appears that they are broken. This is exactly when it is most important to just be with them. I learned this when my older brother became very ill. All my life I

[82] Palmer, P. J. (2000). (p.93) *Let your life speak: Listening for the voice of vocation.* San Francisco: Jossey-Bass.
[83] Palmer, Parker J. "Leading From Within • Center for Courage & Renewal." *Leading from Within.* Center for Courage & Renewal, n.d. Web. 29 May 2015.

had been the sick one; I knew that role well. What I didn't know was how to be on the other side, how to be the person offering consolation. As a person with a disease I had always been frustrated by the pat offers of solace that often came my way. "It will get better." Or the sympathy, "You poor thing to have pain your whole life, how horrible for you!" And the subversive dismissals, "You are so strong; if anyone can handle this you can."

Yet when I became the one needing to respond to the tragic situation that Ned found himself in I found myself falling prey to uttering these very words. I had to literally stop myself at times from letting words slip through my lips that were so similar to the ones I had for so long despised hearing from others. I found myself wanting to offer advice, to say, "It'll get better," to say something, anything to fill the empty space when I was with my brother. I then began to ask myself why I had to do this. When I did I discovered that I wanted to say them to make them true. I wanted to make myself feel better because I knew that my words weren't doing anything to help him. I was trying to protect myself from the reality that my brother's life was in a precarious position, that he may not live to see forty. I realized that seeing someone you love dearly suffering, and being powerless to stop it, is one of the worst things imaginable. I finally understood how hard it had been for my family all those years, that some of the jokes I interpreted as callous were said because the alternative was breaking all the china in the house.

True connection involves compassion. Compassion brings people together and is very different from sympathy, which always divides. Because of my pain over the years I've been on the receiving end of a bucket load of sympathy, and I've become adept at recognizing when a real dose of compassion comes my way.

Here is what sympathy, aka pity, looks like. After fifteen years riding the same mountain bike, I decided it was time to consider a new one. I walked into a bike shop and asked to demo a bike. During the conversation about what I was looking for I told the salesman about the arthritis. I only did this because it was necessary information; I needed to find a bike that rides as smoothly as possible and one that my fused wrists can manage to brake. I instantly regretted mentioning this detail about me, because immediately I heard, "You poor thing! How hard your life must be!" The sales guy went on and on, and I begin to tune him out, trying not to get angry. Hoping to get him back on track I told him, "Actually, my life is not so bad. After all, I'm here looking to buy a mountain bike!"

Sympathy is harmful because it always assumes that a person's situation is negative, and in focusing on the negative it intensifies it. What if I believed all the sympathetic comments that have come my way over the years? I'd believe myself to be a poor thing with a hard life and a tiny, struggling body. How, exactly, does this help me? Sympathy creates a victim, and the idea that the person receiving the sympathy is deficient in some way. A person offering sympathy is able to feel better about his life because, as bad as things sometimes are, at least they don't have the pain, the cleft palate, the divorce, the death in the family. They are forgetting that someday they too will be in a position to receive sympathy. No one goes through life unscathed by pain.

Unlike sympathy, compassion begins with the wish that the other person be free from suffering. A compassionate gesture or comment has within it the desire to be of service and sees suffering as a universal experience. It brings with it the idea that we are all in it together. It is not your pain; it is our pain. When I've been around a compassionate person in a time of need they are willing to sit with me, without judgment, and share my experience, however difficult it has become. During a compassionate encounter with someone I feel lifted and happy, and often we find ourselves laughing. Recently I suffered the loss of a loved one who decided to take his life. In an act of true compassion, my Mom and a friend took me to dinner. As I sat there with a heavy heart looking around and thinking that my loved one would never again feel the wind on his face, I looked at the expression of the two women at the table with me. They hadn't offered any platitudes, or given an explanation about why the suicide happened. They didn't judge the person who did it. Instead we talked, we ordered margaritas, we toasted my loved one, and we laughed. It soothed my soul and made the situation bearable.

There are some other recognizable differences between sympathy and compassion. A sympathetic person assumes that the sufferer is helpless, offers prosaic advice, and escapes as soon as they reasonably can. A compassionate one is there to soothe, is open-minded and genuine, sometimes talks and sometimes has nothing to say, but offers themselves for as long as is needed. The best way to tell if a person is offering compassion or sympathy is to recognize how they make you feel. When I'm being offered sympathy I want to run away, argue, or stand up for myself. I feel diminished and any fear I have about the situation is intensified. Compassion on the other hand, leaves me calmer, stronger, and more full of well-being. Compassion heals.

Rachel Naomi Remen, a physician who has lived with Crohn's disease for most of her life, talks about the difference between service and helping. These are two ways, she says, of approaching life. She says:

> Fundamentally, helping, fixing, and service are ways of seeing life. When you help you see life as weak, when you fix, you see life as broken. When you serve, you see life as whole. From the perspective of service, we are all connected. All suffering is like my suffering and all joy is like my joy. The impulse to serve emerges naturally and inevitably from this way of seeing. In forty years of chronic illness I have been helped by many people and fixed by a great many others who did not recognize my wholeness. All that fixing and helping left me wounded in some important and fundamental ways. Only service heals.[84]

When you are in the presence of someone who is suffering there is only one thing you need to do to help: you need to offer them validation. The words I've most appreciated hearing in all my years living with pain have been, "I'm really sorry you are in so much pain, let me know if I can do anything for you." The action I've most appreciated is companionship. The very act of spending time with me without judgment, commentary, or expectation is worth all the tea in China. There is so much comfort in sharing your life with someone you know won't turn away when the view is less than perfect, when you are a reminder of the vulnerability that comes with being alive. Once the full knowledge that life is a cycle, and eventually we will all be in need, become paramount in one's mind, it becomes easier to be humble enough to be a healing presence for another. The truth is we are all serving each other all the time. Separation is the ultimate illusion, and connection is the ultimate truth.

---

[84] Remen, R. N. (1999). Helping, Fixing, or Serving. *Shambhala Sun*. Retrieved from https://www.uc.edu/content/dam/uc/honors/docs/communityengagement/HelpingFixingServing.pdf

Every day we are presented with so many opportunities to reach out to others. Strangers, family, and friends are all passing through needing to be heard, touched, and loved. So often we move through life trapped in the stories we are telling ourselves, our worries, and our pain. In the midst of this we can easily forget to open our eyes and truly see each other. We can forget that by giving comfort we receive comfort, that by acknowledging the pain of others our own pain is soothed, and that by taking the time to listen to other people's stories we are reminded that although our challenges are unique, the human experience is universal.

When life tries its best to dig a hole and throw us in, it's natural to want to hunker down and keep to yourself. No one wants to be a downer, and sometimes it is so hard to put into words the angst and pain we feel. How do you explain your sadness, anger, fear, or frustration? The truth is, you don't really have to. You just need to climb out of your hole, take a deep breath, and shed the heavy veil that is obscuring your ability to recognize yourself in others. Truly healthy people know that sometimes sharing moments with each other is enough. By showing up and being present with yourself and those around you instead of hiding, no load is too hard to bear.

PAIN

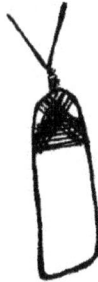

"Kia Kaha, Kia Maia, Kia Manawanui – Be
Strong, Be Persistent, Be Full Of Heart "
-Maori Saying[85]

---

[85] This quote was given to me by my good friend Tipene Pickett, from Auckland, NZ

Pain is an inescapable fact of life. It is the source of endless
suffering and angst. It can seem inescapable. It is a thief,
sucking away a person's life energy, a killer that murders
people who can't find a way to escape it, a demon that seems to
delight in the torture it inflicts. Living with pain is akin to being
a persecuted prisoner. Both generate the same conditions: sleep
deprivation, suffering, extreme discomfort, unpredictability,
feelings of helplessness, and lack of control. Pain is a prison
with invisible walls.

Modern society takes much gratification in its ability to push
pain away. Billions of dollars are spent on prescription
painkillers, billions more on medical surgeries and techniques
that claim to eradicate painful conditions. Pain has become a
pariah; once the word is uttered the next step is always an
attempt to force it to go away. A person living with pain has a
constant reminder that there is something wrong with them. If
the internal cues aren't loud enough there is always the
response from society at large. Admit to being in pain and those
around you will immediately ask what you are doing about it.
Doctors will diagnose you and if they don't find an apparent
physiological reason for your pain they won't hesitate to refer
you to a psychiatrist. A person in pain will spend countless
hours either thinking about their pain, trying to make it go
away, or numbing it. The urgency with which one takes steps to
deaden the pain is a reflection of how the person feels about it.
The more scared you are, the more desperate your actions
become. Once the fear gets the best of you, life becomes a black
hole until all hope has been drained away.

The pain I'm talking about is not just the physical pain we all
have to experience to some degree. It is also the emotional pain
born of life's challenges. Emotional pain is a birthright, one that
can take a lifetime to tame. Inescapable emotional pain can be
deadly; suicide is the tenth leading cause of death in the U.S.,
which isn't even close to the top of the list of high suicide rates
worldwide. When you factor in unreported suicides, pain begins
to loom large. Most people looking inward at their thoughts and
beliefs will find pain and hurt everywhere. Looking outward,
one sees countless ways people use to distract, anesthetize, or
subdue their inner pain. In fact, in many ways the modern
world has formed itself around the pursuit of easy pleasure and
the avoidance of pain. Plentiful food, climate controlled comfort,
cars for everyone to travel at one's whim, easy entertainment
with the click of a remote control, and the ability to literally
close your door and block out the distasteful reminders of

suffering on the street are the hallmarks of modern life. Not that the pursuit of pleasure isn't a worthwhile endeavor, but the denial of an integral part of the experience of living can only result in imbalance and, ironically, ill-health.

"I teach one thing and one thing only: that is, suffering and the end of suffering." –The Buddha[86]

The foundation of Buddhism is the four noble truths. The first noble truth is that life is suffering. This simple statement is enough to turn most Westerners away from Buddhism; who would want to study such a depressing religion, after all? As someone who reached a deep understanding of this idea at a very young age, however, when I first heard these words I thought, "Tell me something I don't know." What I didn't know is that the Buddha actually said that life is dukkha, which has a richer meaning than the word suffering. Dukkha, in its totality, has three categories: pain, called dukkha-dukkha, impermanence or continual change, called viparinama-dukkha, and conditioned states, called samkhara-dukkha, all of which create the conditions for suffering. The four noble truths are like a good-news-bad-news prescription for life.

It's as if the Buddha asked his disciples, "Do you want the bad news or the good news first?" And they answered, "Let's get the bad news over with." What follows the sad truth that life is suffering are three more truths, the causes of suffering and how to move beyond suffering. Now this I could dig into for awhile because anyone who has lived with pain for a length of time knows that pain and suffering aren't simple. They both feel uncomfortable, they both can be triggered easily, and if a person isn't diligent, they both can turn into runaway trains. Depending on a person's choices, however, they both can become the wellspring of true purpose and creativity, creating depth and the origination of wholeness. Eventually, pain and suffering don't even have to be in the same sentence. This takes daily practice and the understanding that most likely this daily practice will last a lifetime. It's a worthwhile endeavor and why digging deeper into the first noble truth can be helpful.

I've never had a day where I've been completely free from pain, or at least one that I can remember. Living with juvenile

---

[86] Rahula, W. (n.d.). Tricycle | Awake in the World. Retrieved from http://www.tricycle.com/new-buddhism/teachings-and-texts/first-sermon-buddha

rheumatoid arthritis since the age of two has made pain my constant companion. Looking back I can break my life up into three distinct categories defined by my relationship to my pain. In short: numbness, anger, and self-acceptance.

My childhood consisted of attempting to hide my pain from others, telling myself no one understood, no one could take it away, and that most people didn't really want to know about it. In reality I couldn't truly hide the pain as it shaped the way I moved and the things I could do, but in my young mind I managed this task well because rarely was it a topic of conversation. People always seemed satisfied with my answer of "fine" whenever I was asked how I was – even my doctor, who was trained to see that this wasn't really true.

I sucked it up and took the Nike sneaker model of "No pain no gain" to heart. I numbed it along with the unruly emotions that came with it. As a result I have large gaps in my childhood memories; luckily I have a best friend I can call to fill in the memory void. I learned to disassociate from my pain, pretending different body parts were separate from me. My stomach was the unruly red-headed step child, my right foot and hand were the little sisters to protect, and my left leg was the oldest child I would always expect the most from and scold if it began to slack. This somehow eased the suffering for me. The act of separating created the illusion that I was okay, even if my pain wasn't. The self-hatred I so often fell into didn't seem so masochistic if the object of my hatred was distanced.

The reaction I'd get from others and the ease with which they were able to ignore the obvious signs of my distress contributed to my muteness on the subject. I remember telling myself as a child, "They can't do anything about it, so why worry them by talking about it?" My go-to answer for how I was doing was "fine," and no one ever challenged it, no matter how much my outward experience contradicted this statement. I didn't know that by holding the burden in, my tiny body was being eaten alive with stress. The triple whammies of lack of opportunity to talk about my pain, the muteness and inexpressibility that I fell into when the rare opportunity did arise, and the ease of denial on the part of the observer created in me a unique web that I wove around the pain which shaped me to the core. This web was there for my survival but like the mishmash of collagen fibers forming the imperfect reproduction of skin that is a scar, this web bound me down in places that I'm only now beginning to discover.

During this time I fed my fragile ego with the knowledge that I had extreme inner strength. I may have been a scrawny kid but on the inside I knew I was stronger than ten rugby players. Unknowingly, this strength became part of my identity, the one thing I knew I was better than anyone at. Pushing through extreme pain became a regular test for me and the better I got at numbing myself, the more proud of myself I became. There were times when I'd go hiking and come back with gaping raw blisters that caused my socks to stick to my heels, and I would have a moment of pride that I hadn't flinched once as I was walking. This was a solo undertaking, one that I shared with no one. My sporadic attempts at putting words to my pain were dismissed, and the truth was that the severity of the pain transcended words, especially words that a child could come up with. So I became an expert at numbing myself and keeping my mouth shut.

Then I experienced a watershed moment. In college I came across an article about chronic pain written by a pain medicine doctor. In it he talked about the emotional aspects of pain, the lack of control, helplessness, and extreme suffering that accompanies the experience of pain. It was as if someone had taken a peek into the deep recesses of my mind and uncovered all of my dark secrets. The façade of interior toughness that I created for myself was just a cover for the anguish I actually felt. He had figured me out and for the first time in my life I broke down. I was in my parents' house and I was sobbing when my Dad came into the room. "What's wrong?" he asked me. Between sobs I showed him the article. He just gave me a bewildered look and I knew I would be alone in this new discovery too.

I spent the next fifteen years of my life battling myself in a different way. Instead of numbing it I began to rage against the pain. My body became the enemy I continued to push out of anger; to spite it I would push it even harder on bad days. I was angry at my doctors, my parents, and myself. My life became a quest to subdue the evil monster that lived inside.

I explored alternative medicine and tried every remedy I came across. I controlled what I ate, what I did, where I lived, and how much I rested. I still hid everything from those around me which meant that nobody could get too close. On the outside I was a happy-go-lucky twenty something with many friends who never knew that I had such a painful disease. I was hiding it in plain sight because the pain had become something to hate, an unsightly stain on my character.

When my body screamed loudly enough I begrudgingly went back to Western medicine and took the drugs that were offered to me. Eventually, these drugs would create a different kind of hell inside and the side effects would get the best of me. I reacted with anger and moved on. I became a shark, always moving because if I stopped I was afraid that I would give up and die. All this anger really was a big lie. It was a mask for the deep anguish that consumed me.

One day I woke up and I was tired. I was tired of fighting my disease, my emotions, and myself. I realized that on a physical level I literally had tried everything I knew of to banish my pain. I finally understood that the answer to leaving pain behind wasn't going to lie in physical manipulation. As Einstein said, you can't solve a problem at the level it was created. So I contemplated the first noble truth, along with some other hard facts about the life I'd created for myself as a reaction to my pain. I finally understood that physical pain may be a condition of my life but the emotional suffering that I had created was optional. Denying, judging, and fighting against the pain in my body did nothing but sustain the civil war going on inside. When I was honest with myself I was able to admit that my thoughts about my pain hurt me more than the pain itself.

A funny thing happens when you take a step back and observe your thoughts. It becomes abundantly clear just how many of them are broken records, which began years ago and are often based on misbeliefs. Once exposed, they begin to lose their power over you. These days, when I find my spirits sinking during a flare-up I watch my thoughts. Inevitably, they will say things like, "Why does this have to happen again, this is my lot in life, I must look like a complete gimp, who'd want to be with someone like me?" I'll look at the runner across the street and think, "He doesn't even appreciate how blessed he is to move without pain, what an ungrateful person."

Sometimes when I examine these thoughts I have to laugh at their absurdity, or how closely they resemble a cliché. "Why me," is definitely a cliché that I have no interest in being associated with. Sometimes though, my harsh thoughts aren't so easy to shake. I have to admit they might just be true. It is quite possible that I'll never be free from pain, that pain is my lot in life.

The question then becomes, okay now what? Not too long ago I pondered this question. What if pain is my lot in life? Does this make my life any less meaningful, any less important, or precious than if I didn't have pain? Yes pain will change my life, but it doesn't have to diminish it in any way.

I'm not a Buddhist, I just like to learn – and Buddhism is a scholarly religion with a framework that works for me. But I'm also a very curious person and an equal opportunity seeker of well-being so when I decided to take a real look at how my pain was perpetuated I had an open mind. I still do, because to me the key to health is mental flexibility. So along with Buddhism, I took in the Toltec wisdom of Don Miguel Ruiz and the spiritual wisdom of teachers like Wayne Dyer, Caroline Myss, and Deepak Chopra. I learned about one of the most famous healers, Jesus. I opened myself up and moved out of my comfort zone at every opportunity. I sought, and I found.

Shamanic ceremonies, meditation, time alone, and prayer became vehicles for self-understanding. They were a way to look into the mirror and finally introduce myself to the real me. When I did, I discovered this about pain: Pain is torture, and living with pain is a huge challenge that takes an immense amount of courage. A life of pain is not an undertaking anyone would wish for him or herself. But pain, like life, especially when it is bad or difficult, will always teach you. The trick is to become an avid student.

James Stockdale was the highest-ranking prisoner of war held in Vietnam. He was once asked which prisoners didn't make it. He replied:

> Oh, that's easy, the optimists. Oh, they were the ones who said, "We're going to be out by Christmas." And Christmas would come, and Christmas would go. Then they'd say, "We're going to be out by Easter." And Easter would come, and Easter would go. And then Thanksgiving, and then it would be Christmas again.

And they died of a broken heart. This is a very important lesson. You must never confuse faith that you will prevail in the end—which you can never afford to lose—with the discipline to confront the most brutal facts of your current reality, whatever they might be. [87]

This became known as the Stockdale Paradox. Taking this paradox to heart and living it enabled me to begin to accept my pain. There is utility in acknowledging the negative aspects of pain while keeping alive the knowledge that at any moment the pain can subside. This isn't false hope; the body is designed to self-heal, which it does twenty-four hours a day, but it does this with its own wisdom and in its own time.

When you are in pain there is a huge incentive to make it go away, but remembering the Stockdale Paradox will prevent you from moving into magical thinking around it. Magical thinking consists of irrational beliefs, especially around causality. The prisoners who died of a broken heart were the ones who set themselves up for disappointment by choosing to believe something that was extremely unlikely. They had no idea when and if they would ever experience freedom again and in telling themselves that freedom was imminent they were creating a hell inside a hell, causing suffering again and again, until it killed them. They weren't able to understand that false hope can be worse than no hope all. False hope is always driven by fear, and in the end actions based on fear will drain hope.

Picture prisoner number one who tells himself, "I'll be out by Christmas, I have to be. Okay, Easter. No, Thanksgiving." Picture his face and demeanor as he lives through each milestone and his wish hasn't been granted. Now prisoner number two. He says, "I'm in a hellacious situation and there is a good chance I will die here. I'm going to be starving, uncomfortable, and physically beaten. But I know I can make it through today, and probably tomorrow. Some people do survive this, so why not me?" When you picture prisoner number two the day after Christmas, Easter, and Thanksgiving, he may be skinnier but he is no less strong. His realistic attitude and strong belief in his ability to survive allow him to do just that.

While I'm on the subject of prison survivors I can't help but return to one of my heroes. Victor Frankl came up with some

---

[87] Collins, James C. "Chapter 4." *Good to Great: Why Some Companies Make the Leap--and Others Don't.* New York, NY: HarperBusiness, 2001. 83-85.

very powerful ideas as a result of his years spent in a Nazi concentration camp, a few of which are very relevant here. In his book Man's Search for Meaning he said:

> Life's meaning is an unconditional one, paralleled by the unconditional value of each person. Just as life remains potentially meaningful under any conditions, even those which are the most miserable, so does the value of each and every person stay with him/ her.

He also said this about suffering:

> Once an individual's search for meaning is successful, it not only renders him happy but also gives him the capability to deal with suffering. Without it you have "give-up it is." Suffering ceases to be suffering the moment it has meaning.[88]

Frankl was also quick to add that unnecessary suffering is masochistic, not heroic.

This point is a linchpin of handling pain well, as well as a skill that takes time to master. Pain, as I said earlier, is a prison without walls, and does torture a person's body. Pain makes you suffer enough. The best thing a person who lives with pain can do for himself is not to compound it. You learn how to do this by feeling the pain instead of numbing it, letting it teach you, and realizing that like all things it will eventually change. This will prevent it from consuming you and killing your soul.

One thing that pain can teach you is how to accept life on life's terms. Life will kick your butt, again and again. It will push you down and show no mercy. It doesn't care who you are or how good you've been. It doesn't punish bad people more than good ones or save those who are deserving. Life is an equal opportunity butt-kicker. The sooner you can accept this reality the sooner you can move into the flow. Throughout my life I've had numerous people, out of compassion, try to make sense of my pain. They've told me, "You're never given more than you can handle, so you must be extremely strong." "Your soul chose this so you can evolve quickly." "You poor thing, a victim of bad genes, you're life must be so hard." I always think, maybe, maybe, maybe, in the end who really cares; does it really matter

---

[88] Frankl, V. (1957). *Mans Search For Meaning*. New York, NY: Pocket Books.

why? Platitudes do nothing for me. The following quote from the stoic philosopher Epictetus does.

"On the occasion of every accident that befalls you, remember to turn to yourself and inquire what power you have for turning it to use." – Epictetus[89]

There is never any use in forcing the natural process of life because life is bigger than any of us will ever know. You can either choose to flow with life or fight it, but fighting it makes you weaker. The metaphor of the surfer always helps me to think of how to flow with the life you have been given. Surfers paddle hard when they need to get through the break, or while getting in position to ride a wave, but in between they are enjoying the feel of the ocean under their board and between their fingers. A surfer who gets impatient and makes his big move too soon will always miss the perfect wave.

All the great teachers emphasize living with less effort; effortless living is an important concept in Taoism, called Wu wei, meaning non-action or non-doing. Lao Tzu in the Tao Te Ching says that those who live in harmony with life (or as he says the Tao), behave in a natural, guileless manner. Trees grow without trying. The sun shines without trying to "do" anything. In fact Lao Tzu says that the goal of spiritual practice for all humans is to learn how to behave naturally. Or as the spiritual teacher of my friend Bob, who I've learned from vicariously, has said, "Live so that your life is no more self-evident than nature." How ironic that the biggest trait we humans have which makes us unique in the world, the ability to invent the new, to strive and achieve grand new circumstances, is the one thing we have to tame. But in certain situations, pain being a perfect example, taming our striving nature is exactly what one must do to minimize suffering.

"You desire to know the art of living, my friend? It is contained in one phrase: make use of suffering." –Henri Frederic Ameil[90]

When you are caught in a riptide the last thing you want to do is to panic. Panic will make you try to swim for shore, which is a sure way to die. Even the best Olympic swimmer in the world wouldn't be able to make it. Instead you have to stave off panic

---

[89] Epictetus. (n.d.). Retrieved from http://izquotes.com/quote/379116
[90] Henri-Frédéric Amiel. (n.d.). Retrieved from http://izquotes.com/quote/280869

and do the unthinkable: swim parallel to the shore until you swim past the riptide, or lie back and let it carry you away from shore until it dissipates. Life challenges can be like a riptide. They can come on quickly and so fiercely no mere mortal will survive resisting them. Resisting life creates anxiety, anxiety feeds fear, and fear causes poor decisions, which in turn induce bad actions. The Buddhists say that the root of all unhappiness is the pursuit of happiness. Don't tell the founding fathers, but the Buddha had a point. The fact is that when you live in pain, the only way to lessen it is to stop trying so hard. Doesn't this ring true for most things in life? Believe me, I know this is another Zen Koan and I don't claim to be a master at it yet, but I am trying, of course in an effortless way!

I do know that someday I will. I know this because even in the midst if the worst pain and anguish I feel I always have access to inner guidance, which sometimes literally becomes a voice that talks to me. As a child I thought of it as my inner scientist and sometimes I still do because it has the tendency during every horrifying situation I've ever been in to say, "Well, isn't this interesting?" This inner voice usually comes out when some joint is ballooning up in front of my eyes and all of a sudden I find that I can no longer walk. Or I'm having a drug reaction and in the span of a few hours I am one big hive. It says, "Kathryn sure is a walking science experiment!" This voice takes on a different tenor when I am in the midst of heartache or grief. In times like this I feel it telling me, "Be glad you are alive and are able to feel." It tells me that life is precious and to be kind to myself. And I do. My inner guidance shows up when I am shaking from pain and wondering if I can take any more.

It was there when I was fourteen and my Mom was literally forcing me into a car to take me back to the hospital because I was still too skinny to be home. I'll never forget that day because I think it actually saved my life. I had escaped from the hospital where I was being kept because I had anorexia and I had been home for a week. Apparently the doctor had told my Mom that I had to come back to the hospital, so she called her friend Mary to escort me because she knew I would resist. I knew something was up when Mary came into the house because of the way they were looking at me and talking in hushed whispers. Quickly they came over and each took me by a scrawny arm saying, "Kathryn, you have to go back to the hospital." In that instant my heart broke. I felt utterly betrayed.

It was as if I was being kidnapped, which in a way I was. I felt this because for me the anorexia was never about being skinny, it was about feeling completely out of control over my disease and my life. Instead of involving me and explaining their decision about my destiny, they both had decided for me. Looking back I completely understand just how dire my situation was, and from their perspective this was the best way to handle things. In that moment though, I felt my heart stop. The anorexia had affected my heart, which is how I ended up hospitalized in the first place and my inner voice told me to stop because I was about to have a heart attack. I asked my Mom for a minute and I sat down in a chair until I could feel my body calming itself. Then I asked for something to eat. I needed my strength to go back to the hospital. To this day I know that if my inner voice hadn't kicked in and instructed me I would have died.

This inner guidance has another aspect; it can bring peace. There is a peaceful feeling inside that can always see the beauty in every situation. It is the knowledge that my life, as James Blunt says, is brilliant, like a gemstone – even the rough edges. My inner peace holds me close and considers me precious, belonging to life and necessary to the world, and in my darkest hours it soothes me. Some would call this God, Spirit, or intuition. I don't have a name. For me this aspect to my life is ultimately beyond words. I do know that I am eternally grateful for my ability to feel and hold onto my inner wisdom and the peace it brings, because without it I would not be able to survive the amount of pain I've had to endure.

If you don't know what I'm talking about, you may need to dig for it, but I promise it will be there. Consider the following excerpt from the book *Let Your Life Speak: Listening to the Voice of Vocation*, by Parker J. Palmer. In this passage he is describing an Outward Bound experience he once had. He was attempting a roped-in rock climb, meaning he was climbing under his own power but was wearing a harness that was attached to a rope that held him. As he was afraid of heights, he was scared witless:

> Parker, is anything wrong? To this day, I do not know where my words came from, though I have twelve witnesses to the fact that I spoke them. In a high, squeaky voice I said, "I don't want to talk about it." "Then," said the second instructor, "it's time that you learned the Outward Bound motto. "Oh, keen, I thought.

"I'm about to die, and she's going to give me a motto!"
But then she shouted ten words I hope never to forget,
words whose impact and meaning I can still feel: "If you
can't get out of it, get into it!"[91]

If you can't get out of it, get into it. This is a sentence that
makes one pause. We all experience times in our life when
circumstances are difficult and can feel inescapable. You may
never have been trapped on a rock face, too afraid to move up
or down, but figuratively life will take you to this rock face at
some point. The best thing anyone can do when they find
themselves here is to stop struggling against and start moving
toward. Not toward the trouble they find themselves in, or
toward yet another possible solution, but toward the true
meaning and lessons found within the experience.

This may still seem like Greek, but if you can stay with me, I
will try to explain. If you remember, resilience is the ability to
bounce back from challenges, not unscathed, but stronger,
better, healthier, and wiser than before. People who do this are
able to at some point surrender to the experience, and when
they do they naturally go inside. In the book *Deep Survival,
Who Lives, Who Dies, and Why*, author Laurence Gonzales tells
the story of a young woman who was the sole survivor of a
plane crash in the Amazon. She and a handful of adult
passengers were flying in a small plane that crashed, and she
remembers looking out the window as they were plummeting to
the ground thinking that the jungle canopy looked like a bunch
of big green mushrooms. She wasn't imagining a fiery death, or
bemoaning her fate; she was feeling awe at the beauty in
nature. She was moving into the experience, not fighting
against it. There are numerous stories of POWs who, as they
were on a forced march to a prison, were able to look around
and marvel at the blue sky, the monkeys chirping in the trees,
or the verdant green of the jungle flora. Like this young girl
they went on to not only survive their experience, but also to
transcend it. There is beauty in everything and inner wisdom is
the only way to grow eyes that see it. To get there you have to
dig deep and mine through your fears.

We all know a few people who go through life under the guise of
the walking wounded. Maybe you've been one. These people
walk around with their wounds on their sleeve, so much so that

---

[91] Palmer, P. J. (2000). (p.84) *Let your life speak: Listening for the voice of vocation.*
San Francisco: Jossey-Bass.

after awhile their wounds walk into the room before they do. When you think of these people the first thing that comes to your mind is their wound. Then you'll wonder what part of the wound you'll have to talk about when you see them next. Their wounds excite and impassion them; if they were sexually abused they will know about every rape case hitting the news, and every pedophile that has recently been released from prison. If they have a physical ailment they will be eager to tell you just why they can't do the particular activity you suggested, however benign. Their wound psychically infects them to the point that they and the wound become one. They are the definition of a masochist, deriving pleasure from their tormented state.

How does one become a member of this sad group of people? Is it because they like the attention? Is it because they receive sympathy from the people around them? Or is it something else, something deeper? Perhaps, the deeper reason for this lifestyle choice is that they never went into their wound, as the Outward Bound motto extolls. They never moved past the fear that consumed them during their trauma. They never knew that if they scratched the surface, inside their scarred body there is a deep, unending well that soothes even the greatest pain.

The wounds that pain inflicts on a person can be insidious. If you aren't careful your pain will overtake your identity, and you will forever walk through the world wounded. In order for you to walk away from your wound you have to always realize that your wound isn't you, it is something that happened to you, or perhaps something that is happening to you. Your wound, your pain, quite possibly has shaped who you are and who you will become, but it doesn't have to taint your core. In fact, if you move into it, you will find that, just like a broken bone that heals stronger than before, so can your wounded self.

"I am not a strong woman, I am a woman of strength."
–Edith Eva Eger[92]

Dr. Edith Eva Eger was sixteen when she was brought with her parents to Auschwitz. Her parents were sent to the gas chambers; as a young, strong woman she was kept alive. Dr.

[92] Sherwood, B. (2009). The Dancer and the Angel of Death. In *The Survivors Club: The Secrets and Science that Could Save Your Life.* New York, NY: Grand Central Publishing.

Joseph Mengele wanted someone around who could dance for him, so she was sent to perform for the notorious angel of death:

"I closed my eyes and I pretended that I was far away from Auschwitz and the music was Tchaikovsky, and I was dancing the Romeo and Juliet in the Budapest Opera House."
– Dr. Edith Eva Eger[93]

Throughout her years at Auschwitz, Eva was able to see herself through the eyes of a third person, to see her situation from outside herself so that she could survive:

> I went from feeling myself victimized by our keepers to the realization that I quite possibly had the inner resources to outlast them. That somehow I could match their collective decision to eliminate us as human beings and Jews with my determination to live.[94]

Eva is the perfect example of a person who was able to handle extreme life challenges with grace. Pain, disease, and extreme hardship create unique opportunities for personal growth and wisdom, for discovering true gratitude and uncovering the innate resilience that we are all born with. Pain is crucial in making us real, humbling us to the point that we are able to feel true compassion, and understanding that we really are all connected. Pain, instead of closing us down, will open us up if we are able to do one thing: stop saying "take it away," and start saying "show me the way."

I once heard a graduation speech given by Maria Shriver. One thing she said stood out: life is a marathon, not a race. These words changed me. Since the day I heard them I've been able to reign in my emotions when I get frustrated with the pace my life is taking, or with my perceived lack of improvement when my pain has stayed bad for a prolonged period of time. Maria's words help me to remember that big changes come through small steps, literally one step at a time. It's true that we never know when our number is up. I could get hit by a Mack truck tomorrow, but even if I did I know that it wouldn't help to look

---

[93] Eger, E. E. (2015, March 18). I Don't Know What I Would Have Been Without Auschwitz. Retrieved from http://www.huffingtonpost.com/edith-eva-eger/i-dont-know-what-i-would-_b_6895940.html
[94] Edith, E. (n.d.). There are No Crises, Only Transitions. Retrieved from http://www.dreee.com/downloads/PressRelease_20050901.pdf

at life in any other way. Each step can take you where you need to go, and you never know what you'll find along the path. Choosing your steps, however, can be challenging. The age of information that we find ourselves in is a double-edged sword. It brings with it tremendous opportunity to educate oneself, but the sheer volume of it can also paralyze a person who is trying to figure out how best to help herself when she is faced with pain or disease. This is especially true when your previous attempts to help yourself haven't been successful – when your life, despite your best efforts, just isn't getting better.

When circumstances look the most bleak true courage emerges. The ability to endure pain or adversity with fortitude and strength is extremely hard. When your choices thus far have appeared to keep you stuck, how do you find the internal resources to keep going? There are no easy answers to this, but there is inspiration from those who've gone before.

Every book about extreme survival says the same thing about what it takes to be a survivor. You need to keep your wits about you, accept your present circumstance by not struggling against it or moving into denial, believe that you will prevail in the end, and then act on this belief. My life history has taught me these skills well. Rheumatoid arthritis can at times be savage. It can hit hard and fast, completely obliterate your ability to function, and cause pain beyond the imagination. But it also has an ironic quality to it as well. It can disappear almost as suddenly as it came, sometimes without warning. So, over the years when I've told myself, "This too shall pass," I know I'm not deluding myself. This doesn't make the physical situation that I'm in any easier, but it does lift the mental torment that accompanies it. It also allows me to think more clearly about what I need to do next to feel better.

When you are in pain or dealing with a life challenge, not struggling against it is paramount. It is the only way you will be able to ever transcend your situation, the only way you can master any of the other survival skills. Letting go of the struggle is the fundamental life skill one needs to be proficient at any of the others. It may also the hardest to master, something I know well as it continues to be a daily practice for me.

Not struggling against pain doesn't seem natural. After all, pain is an uncomfortable state that encourages resistance. Modern society teaches us that pain should be eradicated; life challenges are an aberration requiring immediate fixing, and often those who are experiencing physical pain or other life challenges are to blame in some way. This worldview does nothing but inhibit a person's ability to fully become whole and healed. Instead, the true path to healing is in remembering this quote from Parker J. Palmer: *Wholeness does not mean perfection; it means embracing brokenness as an integral part of life.*[95] Once you understand this truism you can more easily stop running away from your shadow and start living with heart. The brokenness, the pain, and the challenge are just as important, just as valuable, just as lovable as the pretty, easy-to-show parts of yourself.

It's crucial to take this to heart; opening yourself up to living within the experience of life without judging it is really the only way you will ever be able to transcend the painful experiences that life will inevitably dole out. It took me years and years of feeling disgust and revulsion when I looked at my swollen joints before I finally realized that those swollen joints were working hard for me every day, allowing me to function despite my sometimes unreasonable demands on them. The crooked fingers and fused wrists that I try so hard to hide may prevent me from being a hand model, but they hold up just fine even when I'm submitting them to a long, pounding, mountain bike ride. The very aspects of myself that I've wasted so much energy trying to repress are the parts that have taught me extreme fortitude, resilience, and courage. The broken, unsightly parts of myself have been a catalyst for exposing my shadow as I've internally and externally raged against them, but when I was finally able to look at my shadow in the mirror, just like the Wizard of Oz, it became less powerful.

Not judging your pain doesn't in any way minimize the hard realities it creates. My pain changes my personality as it sucks my life energy. People who know me become acquainted with two different people. When the pain is bad I am quieter, less spontaneous, more rigid in my lifestyle, and more anxious as my faith that I'll be okay is tested. When things are really bad I can appear like a timid wallflower. The other side to this split personality comes out when the pain lifts. This is when I'm smiling all the time as I suck the juice out of life and savor every moment. I'm outside a lot, enjoying the feel of a body that moves with less hesitation. I am more social, and I am much

---

95 A quote by Parker J. Palmer. (n.d.). Retrieved from http://www.goodreads.com/quotes/1225465-wholeness-does-not-mean-perfection-it-means-embracing-brokenness-as

more outgoing. When I feel good, the unconscious urge to hide is no longer there and my self-esteem is fully intact.

Over the years it has been an enormous challenge to remember the real me when it is in hibernation for years on end as my pain takes over. Not allowing the pain to break me down to the point of no return has been a nearly insurmountable task. I've seen many people throughout my career as an occupational therapist who aren't able to do this, and they appeared defeated in every way. Their speech, posture, actions and isolated lifestyles all reflect just how far down the rabbit hole of despair they have gone. Pain will either swallow you whole or make you whole. Ultimately it's your choice whether to hurt or to heal, one that you have to make time and again, until you know for certain that the pain has strengthened your resolve enough that it won't ever defeat you.

"Affliction is the wholesome soil of virtue, where patience, honor, sweet humility, and calm fortitude, take root and strongly flourish." –David Mallet[96]

I have a deeper relationship to pain than to anything or anyone else in my life. If my pain were a person I'd describe this mighty waif as mercurial. Sometimes Pain acts like an irate Tinker Bell. Pain can also resemble the devil itself. Pain is like a lover that I try to forget yet keeps coming to visit me at night while I'm dreaming. I attempt to placate Pain, and break up with it in a dignified and loving manner. I gently tell Pain that it's time we move on from each other. I've grown past it and I need to use my precious energy on other relationships. I really, truly appreciate all that it has taught me, the strength and resolve it has helped me to grow, but if it continues to occupy my life it will consume me. I plead with Pain, and tell Pain that No, my life purpose is not to live with such a demanding character as you; I am supposed to love another. But Pain doesn't listen to my pleading. So instead Pain and I have come to live together, like an old married couple weary of each other but in it for the duration. We have a lot of private jokes. Sarcastically I tell it how much I enjoy being a walking science experiment and that I'm getting seasick from all the ups and downs it makes me ride through.

---

[96] David Mallet is an American Singer/Songwriter David Mallet quote. (n.d.). Retrieved from http://www.brainyquote.com/quotes/quotes/d/davidmalle204308.html

Only recently have I realized that what I thought was an illusion was in fact true. In my hopelessness I'd convinced myself that I was kidding myself to believe that I'd ever be okay. Now I know that I was always okay. I am okay. Sometimes the truth is simple, and for me the truth is that pain may be mandatory but the angst that so often comes with it is optional. The familiar feeling of dread can be lifted by moving away from the isolation that pain can so easily bring, and moving into honesty with myself and the people who surround me. Instead of cushioning others from the reality of my life I've begun to show them who I really am, pain and all. I'm finding that the elephant in the room isn't so big and awkward anymore.

So now, as I walk through life, I ask myself often, "Who do you want to be?" The answer is where I place my focus, where I choose to stand, and it empowers me. My experiences have made my life richer, and the meaning I have taken from them help to propel me into a future that will continue to fascinate. This I know: Pain and I are in for a wild ride.

Like death and taxes, pain is an inevitable part of life. Without the ability to handle pain well, you will never be truly healthy. Pain uncovers a person's shadow, tempting each one of us, like a demon, to fall into victimhood. It condemns some of us to a life of attempting to numb or run away from what we don't want to feel. But pain can also be an open door to a new way of living, with gentle discipline, awareness, an open heart, and true compassion. Fredrich Nietzche famously said, "That which does not destroy, strengthens." Severe pain is a catalyst for change, change opens the door to growth, growth brings wholeness, and wholeness equals health. In the end, pain teaches us that our true self is not the anxious, critical, or fearful person who frowns when we look in the mirror, but the one inside that is always fighting for our life

SPIRIT

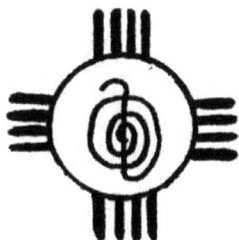

"I will not forget you. I have you carved in the palm of my hand."

-Isaiah 49:15

A few years ago I was teaching a class to a group of Veterans about creating a balanced life. I had spent a lot of time preparing the material and had a handout with a picture of a wheel for everyone. Each spoke in the wheel represented a different area of life: work, hobbies, time with loved ones, exercise, sleep, etc. I began talking about the wheel when a voice from the corner of the room piped up. The voice said, "What about spirituality?" Chagrined, I realized I had completely left out the thread that weaves through every aspect of life. Something so important, yet so invisible, that sometimes we forget to include it when we are talking about life or health.

Say the word spirituality and people have a myriad of associations. When I posed the question, "What do you think of when you hear the word spirituality?" to my friends and associates, I heard answers like:

"Energy, peace, serenity, strength, inner life."

"The way you connect with life."

"Connection to my authentic self, and a peaceful knowing that I am connected to every living being, animal, and bit of nature on this planet."

"To live in your heart, not in your head."

The answers were as unique as a snowflake; each was made of the same ingredients, but also completely individual. The common thread to all of them is a connection to the sacred, the unseen divine force that connects everything and everyone. Hindu monk Swami Vedananda said this when explaining spirituality: "What spirituality is can only be felt, it can't be defined, all definitions are limited and spirituality is unlimited."[97] Spirituality is experiential; it has to be experienced rather than explained.

A small minority of people can live denying the existence of the spiritual. They say that the emotional wellbeing one feels when contemplating the connectedness of all things is just a state of mind, a psychological or emotional response that has its underpinnings in physiology. They are quick to react against

---

[97] Swami Vedananda - What Is Spirituality? (n.d.). Retrieved from
http://www.spiritube.com/swami-vedananda-what-is-spirituality-video_e161947d4.html

accepting an unknown force greater than humans can understand and their search for rational answers becomes a replacement for the dogma of religion. The famous atheist Richard Dawkins once remarked, "I am against religion because it teaches us to be satisfied with not understanding the world."[98]

I feel that these rationalists protest a bit too much against spirituality and I have to wonder why. Their lack of true inquiry about the nature of a spiritual life means that they never understand that spirituality is a verb, not a noun. It doesn't breed complacency. In fact, quite the opposite; it is a call to action, a commitment to self and others, a hard road to take. As humans we like to categorize, pigeonhole others, and explain everything. We forget that some things are completely individual and beyond words. This is Spirituality.

"Spirit is an invisible force made visible in all of life."
–Maya Angelou[99]

Connection with spirit is embedded in our DNA. Since the dawn of humans spirit has been interwoven into life; it is only the past few hundred years that modern civilization created a separate category for it. This separation was a specific event that is traced to Rene Descartes, founder of modern philosophy. In order to get bodies for dissection and allow scientists to proceed with their inquiries without being burned at the stake for heresy, Descartes agreed he wouldn't have anything to do with the soul, mind, or emotions if he could have the physical realm. This deal has influenced culture and modern thinking ever since.

In the bubble of modern living, however, we forget from where we came. This blind spot has harmed us, especially when it comes to health and healing. Unlike modern medicine, indigenous cultures include spirituality in the healing process. Spirituality is integral in the process of healing because all things are connected and physical health is an expression of the spirit. Indigenous cultures understand life in the context of spirit; harmony in thoughts, actions, and a person's relationship to their inner and outer world is necessary for true health to be restored.

---

[98] "Richard Dawkins Quote." BrainyQuote. Xplore, n.d. Web. 29 May 2015.
[99] Maya Angelou. (n.d.). Retrieved from http://izquotes.com/quote/321174

If we can't see it, smell it, touch it, or measure it, how do we know it is there? How does one begin to approach the experience of spirituality? Deepak Chopra says that experiencing spirituality involves four aspects: being, feeling, thinking, and doing. Being is found in self-reflection, quieting the mind, being present with oneself in the world, and meditation. Feeling is discovered through relationships, specifically love, leading to connection, communion, and intimacy with those who share our lives. Thinking is the intellectual quest for the way the universe works and a thoughtful approach to see the connections throughout the web of life, the creative aspect of the world. Finally, doing involves service: service to self and to others, healing yourself and all those around you. Altruistic service is service to the spirit, which can be felt. The cornerstone of spirituality, however, is getting the mind out of the way. The mind keeps us separate and is unable to fully grasp the potential of the spirit.

Every day our bodies remind us of their limitations. We can only see, hear, and feel so well. We need water and food regularly, air almost constantly, and we need to maintain a certain temperature and pH in order for our bodies to function adequately. Sometimes, though, we are pushed beyond our limits and survive. How do we do this? Where does the strength come from to survive seemingly un-survivable situations? Victor Frankl said:

> As a professor in two fields, neurology and psychiatry, I am fully aware of the extent to which man is subject to biological, psychological and sociological conditions. But in addition to being a professor in two fields I am a survivor of four camps – concentration camps that is – and as such I also bear witness to the unexpected extent to which man is capable of defying and braving even the worst conditions conceivable. [100]

I still remember reading Eli Wiesel's book *Night*, in junior high school. In the book he describes his experiences as a youngster living in two concentration camps during WWII. It made me wonder, "How can a person live on watery gruel and a hunk of bread for years at a time, doing manual labor outside in extreme conditions, during the brutal cold of winter and the searing hot of summer? Sleeping head to foot on wooden planks at night with no blanket?" Sadly, the concentration camps

---

[100] Frankl, V. (1957). *Mans Search For Meaning*. New York, NY: Pocket Books.

during WWII were only one example of the many ways humans have conspired to torture each other. Populations have been persecuted in agonizing ways and unimaginable conditions have brought them to the brink of death. But many survive. How is this possible?

I believe that the immense power of the spirit can take over when the body is about to give up. I believe this because I've experienced it, time and again in my life. Throughout my life I've had the opportunity to experience pain so severe I've wanted to chew off my own hand to distract myself. As a very young person my pain was so severe that anorexia became a respite for me. Starvation took away the energy my body needed to create arthritis, and as I shrank, my pain was better. The discomfort from constant hunger and sitting on bones with no flesh to pad them was easy to endure in comparison. However, this led to an inner struggle: Did I want to save my life by gaining weight, only to return to a body that tortured me? Impossibly, the logical, the sane response would have been "No!" What kind of life would I have to look forward to?

I remember all too well my state of mind back then. I was living in Columbia-Presbyterian hospital because I was so frail I had to be monitored 24/7. Columbia-Presbyterian had an arts and crafts room for kids who were hospitalized for a long time and I spent most of my days there making endless bracelets and plaster figurines. This room saved my life because it kept my hands busy as my spirit was able to kick in and infuse hope into the predicament of my life. As I busily worked away, inside I was deepening my spiritual resolve.

One day I found myself staring out the window of the arts and crafts room listening to the John Waite song, "Missing You," on my headphones. I was staring through the sterile, quadruple-paned window that wouldn't open to bring fresh air to my face, nine floors above all the people purposefully walking on the streets below, and I felt utterly lost. In my ears I heard John Waite sing about his frozen, desperate heart that was losing it's fight in the midst of lost love.

I was too young to understand the meaning that John Waite was trying to convey, but the meaning I gleaned for myself was all too true. I knew I was losing the fight for my life and I wasn't sure what the outcome would be. I was utterly alone in the world, in my experience, and even though I had doctors, parents, family, and friends who desperately wanted me to live they had no true understanding of the life they were condemning me to.

The decision about whether to live or die was mine to make. In the end, life was my choice because although I didn't understand why I had to suffer so intensely, I didn't want to give up. I felt that I would grow to discover the fruits of the indomitable spirit I was developing; perhaps impossible healing was possible. Although I wasn't able to articulate this to myself at the time, I knew that every stage of life, whether easy or difficult, is necessary to the revelation of true identity and I had to live to find out what that might be. Somehow, even though I was a religious neophyte with very little spiritual education to rely upon, I knew that even if I felt isolated from those around me I was never outside the divine. I was, as Caroline Myss says, developing a soul strong enough that it couldn't be scared.

I had to visit the brink of death to decide to live. The decision only came after I got in touch with my spirit. I've come to believe that God, the Divine, only brings us what is most beneficial for the growth of our soul. These lessons may be terrifying and arduous, but they are necessary, because in the end they bring us inspiration. The real work, however, isn't surviving difficult times. It is honoring the inspiration you receive when going through them. We are all inspired at one time or another but only a few of us seriously listen and take action that respects the inner wisdom we receive. This is because inner guidance will inevitably tell us to create change and when we are going through challenges all we want is comfort, not more uncertainty. Often the changes we are called to make are difficult to explain to those around us. Explaining your choices to others by saying, "I'm following my intuition, my inner voice, or my higher self," can result in blank stares or logical arguments as to why you should stay right where you are. They can even be met with anger, derision, or contempt. This is when a person can remember these words, an adaptation of the Paradoxical Commandments, written by Kent M. Keith.

> People are often unreasonable and self-centered. Forgive them anyway. If you are kind, people may accuse you of ulterior motives. Be kind anyway. If you are honest, people may cheat you. Be honest anyway. If you find happiness, people may be jealous. Be happy anyway. The good you do today may be forgotten tomorrow. Do good anyway. Give the world the best you

have and it may never be enough. Give your best anyway. For you see, in the end, it is between you and God. It was never between you and them anyway.[101]

When we live with reverence for the sacred aspects of life we are less likely to be swayed by popular opinion and more likely to be kind, because we live with the knowledge of just how connected all things are. Spiritual inquiry may call one to ask, "What if I am part of a bigger organism, and have a purpose for the health of the whole?" This question causes us to become more receptive to guidance and less rigid, to learn to participate, not to control. We find ourselves wanting not only to empower ourselves but to empower others as well. Live as though you are just one strand in the web of life and you won't hold so tightly to your beliefs or your story. Your physical body and life circumstances mirror what your soul needs to work on, not just for yourself but for the whole. Remaining open to understanding the lessons that life has to offer is the only way people can heal themselves and their lives. Over time, challenges may not disappear but they will stop triggering you to suffer. Pain is inevitable, but suffering can be optional.

"If I want you to be the least bit different then you become an object in my mind instead of a subject in my heart. Where is the healing there, it's just separation." –Stephen Levine[102]

How many times I have heard people who claim to take their spirituality seriously tell me, "I only want to be around people on a spiritual path. I have no time for people who just don't get it." I hold my tongue but I know that they are missing the point. We are all on a spiritual path. And we are all called to honor the individual path that each one of us is on. Spirituality has as many meanings as there are people defining it or denying it, and just as many paths as there are people. You may look at me and see all the things I'm doing wrong and I may look at you and see the same, but in the end we are both right for walking down our individual roads, and both wrong for judging the way

---

[101] This quote is an adaptation of The Paradoxical Commandments, written by a 19 year old Harvard University Student named Kent M. Keith in 1968. You can see the original here: http://www.paradoxicalcommandments.com/origin.html

Keith, K. M. (n.d.). The Mother Teresa Connection - Dr. Kent M. Keith. Retrieved from http://www.kentmkeith.com/mother_teresa.html

[102] Mishlove, J. (n.d.). THE NATURE OF HEALING with STEPHEN LEVINE. Retrieved from http://www.intuition.org/txt/levine.htm

the other walks. The most important thing anyone can do for himself is to stop judging and start being patient with the process because it is a long and winding road. The rockier the road becomes, the more you will be directed.

If I went out to lunch with three of my friends and after lunch a fourth friend came up to us and asked us to describe the restaurant, he would get four very different answers. One person may concentrate on the noise level, the food, the staff, another may notice the paintings on the wall and the color of the concrete floors, a third may have seen the pretty flowers on each table, and so on. But none of us would have the same answer. This material world, which seems so obvious to the naked eye, isn't so obvious once you scratch the surface.

Sure the sky is blue, the table is round, the wind is strong, the dog has four legs; most of us can agree on that. But a color-blind person doesn't see the blue sky, she sees a gray sky. A hard of hearing person may be convinced they are alone in a room when in actuality there are two people behind them. Someone with acute eyesight may see the hummingbird in the tree while the rest of us are oblivious to its gentle presence. Eyewitness accounts don't hold the weight they once had during court cases because study after study has demonstrated just how unreliable they are. If our experience of the dense, material world is so hard to agree upon, think about just how challenging the task of describing the spiritual world is. Especially in cultures where true spirituality has been brushed aside for centuries; in the modern age spirituality has become the red-headed step-child in the family of rational inquiry.

Anyone who opens his heart to a spiritual life will find a deep well to draw from. The experiences found in this well are deeply personal and can feel just as real as the chair you sit on. But because of the intimacy of each person's perception of spirit I would never presume to tell anyone what his spirituality should be like; instead what I can do is tell you what spirituality is for me. Spirituality has challenged me more than anything in my life. Pain I can easily understand on a physical level. There is an explanation for why I live with pain that has to do with inflammation, changes to the structure of my joints, and hypersensitive nerve endings. What I wrestle with is whether there is a deeper meaning to the pain, and if so, what that meaning may be. Did my soul choose pain to help me evolve? Did God give me pain to bring me closer to him?

I do know that illness has been my spiritual guru. It has humbled me so that I never get on a high horse. It has helped me to realize my gifts and my inner strength. It has scared me so much that nothing much scares me anymore. It has taught me how to love and share compassion and it has shown me well the value of living comfortably with uncertainty. My pain has made it abundantly clear that as much as we seek to understand, in the end most of life is beyond our comprehension; that the only way to live well is to enjoy the mystery. Live with the questions but never stop trying to find answers, do the best you can without judging yourself when your best doesn't seem good enough, and know that eventually at least some things will make sense.

My relationship with my spirituality is rocky because sometimes the direction I receive isn't what I want to hear and sometimes no direction is forthcoming when I'm so desperate I'd do anything I was guided to do. For me spirituality is very real, and permeates my daily life. I don't confine it to a specific day for worship or a specific time for meditation. It is with me always. The pain has been a vehicle for touching spirit because it makes me long to leave my body, and over the years this longing has borne fruit. William Buhlman, author of Secret of the Soul and a pioneer in out-of-body experiences, says that spiritual experience is transcending the limits of the physical body. It is the core element of all religions; it is referenced throughout the Bible, the basis for Islam, and one element that connects all religious mystics. Once you strip away the physical façade, the language of being human, you are able to connect with the creative force of the universe.

My experience leads me to believe this is true. I feel a connection to the universal consciousness some call energy and it guides me through what I call my higher self. I can access it a variety of ways: deliberately during meditation, through my work with my good friend who is an energy healer, or the use of muscle testing, and it comes to me regularly in my dreams. My dreams don't pay attention to time. Sometimes they tell me my future, and sometimes they help to heal my past; they are always wiser than my rational, conscious mind. They are a connection to spirit. My spirituality brings me reverence for the experience of life and the ability to endure even the most painful times of my life because I know that I am necessary and I'm curious to see what will come next. When my prayers aren't answered I lay down my load at the feet of the divine and trust that at least some of my burden will be lifted. It always is.

"Take the riskiest path you can find. Keep your attention in the present time. Carry no extraneous baggage. Forgive everybody you can. Pray daily. Manage your spirit with integrity and honor. Keep your personal honor code and never break it. Everything matters." –Caroline Myss[103]

This response to how to manage one's spirit is my favorite quote by Caroline Myss. She also says that the soul always knows what to do to heal itself. Our only job is to quiet the mind. This takes courage but reaps great reward. I've found that honoring my spirit raises the bar on every aspect of my life. It takes me out of the victim role and has made me a maverick patient as I respect my inner wisdom just as much as the educated advice of the health professionals I seek out. It guides me on whom to seek out for assistance and gives me the strength to first go inside myself instead of always looking outside for the answers I seek. It's made me responsible for myself and keeps me in my integrity regardless of my external circumstances. It has led me to take everything and nothing personally. And most important, it has taught me the value of forgiveness, both of myself and others. I believe that the purest, most spiritual, and loving people may have the hardest hurdles to overcome, perhaps because the hurdles always bring with them the opportunity to reach into the divine. And deep in my heart I know that true health and deep spirituality always go hand in hand.

---

[103] Toms, M. (n.d.). Caroline Myss News | In The Media | News Detail. Retrieved from http://www.myss.com/news/media/adetail.asp?i=18

WISDOM

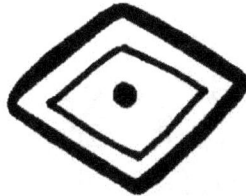

"I salute the light within your eyes where the whole Universe dwells. For when you are at that center within you and I am that place within me, we shall be one."

Crazy Horse, Oglala Lakota Sioux
(circa 1840-1877)[104]

[104] Horse, C. (n.d.). ONLY THE BEST NATIVE AMERICAN INDIAN QUOTATIONS Modern & Traditional Words of Guidance... Retrieved from http://www.californiaindianeducation.org/inspire/traditional

WISE PEOPLE:

- Live Free from Judgment
- Exude Peace; people feel peaceful when they are with them
- Are Genuinely Happy; they Laugh and Smile a lot
- Are Steadfast with Kindness
- Have Personal Integrity, and a Personal Honor Code that they don't break
- Have the ability to change perspective
- Choose Love not fear
- Practice Wise Speech
- Are always seeking, yet always content
- Remain open, cultivating beginner's mind
- Are Humble
- Cultivate True Friendship
- Value Truth
- Know that True Abundance is having what you need when you need it

Wisdom is the Holy Grail that can come with age, but it is not a certainty. Each of us has the choice whether to turn the experiences and knowledge that we gain throughout our lives into the insights that create wisdom. Gaining wisdom will forever shift the way you approach your life because wisdom brings changes in perspective and a deeper understanding of the world. Wisdom is a virtue, one that people will be drawn to as they seek their own deeper truth. A wise person is a magnet for others seeking wisdom. The irony is that the wiser one becomes, the deeper you understand, as Socrates said, *"There is only one thing that I know, and I know that I know nothing."*[105]

Do you need wisdom in order to have a healthy life? Without hesitation I can say yes, and I can also say that a lifelong quest to acquire wisdom is a valiant one. Wisdom will make you a better person and more valuable. The rewards of wisdom last a lifetime and build upon themselves. Open the door to a piece of wisdom and you will never go back. How does one become wise? Are there steps to follow; is there a manual for the wise? Is it a clear path or a circuitous route? Is wisdom the same for one and all or is wisdom personal?

The answer is yes. My own search for wisdom has led me to where I stand now, with a better understanding of the wisdom of my own life.

The older you get, the more you have the opportunity to witness the spectrum of human behavior. Eventually, the good, the bad, and the ugly will reveal themselves to you in some form, sometimes over and over. If you pay attention long enough you will discover a few things, including the fact that there are commonalities to what people do to create misery in their lives. Here are my top three: letting the ego take control of identity, taking emotions too seriously, and rigid thinking or dogmatism. There are also commonalities to what people do to create happiness: mental flexibility, compassion, a curious attitude, and the ability to persevere in the face of enduring challenges.

Have you ever compared the words of prophets like Jesus, or Muhammad with the religions that they begat? It's always striking to me that dogma is the inevitable result of such divinely inspired people. Dogmatism, according to the free dictionary, is an authoritative principle, belief, or statement of

---

[105] "I Know That I Know Nothing." Wikipedia. Wikimedia Foundation, n.d. Web. 29 May 2015.

ideas or opinion, especially one considered to be absolutely true. Sounds benign, correct? Now consider the rest of the definition: "Arrogant, stubborn assertion of opinion or belief, a statement of a point of view as if it were an established fact, or the use of a system of ideas based upon insufficiently examined premises."[106] Not so benign anymore. Read the following quotes from these two great men, and then reflect on the religions that claim to follow their teachings.

"Be steadfast, enjoin kindness, avoid ignorance, and bear with patience whatever befalls you." -The Quran 31:17

"The most excellent jihad is the conquest of the self."[107]

"Even as the fingers of the two hands are equal, so are human beings equal to one another. No one has any right, nor any preference to claim over another. You are brothers." [108]

"There's no 'ifs' among believers. Anything can happen." –Jesus (Mark 9:23)

"Do to others whatever you would like them to do to you. This is the essence of all that is taught in the law and the prophets. (Matthew 7:12)

"And so I tell you, keep on asking, and you will receive what you ask for. Keep on seeking, and you will find. Keep on knocking, and the door will be opened to you. For everyone who asks, receives. Everyone who seeks, finds. And to everyone who knocks, the door will be opened. (Luke 11:9-10)

These words are not prescriptive. Rather, they are guidance for those who are seekers. The religious dogma that followed them has little to do with the personal quest for enlightenment that the prophets were calling for. Why then, do people so easily fall under the spell of dogmatic thinking? I'm not claiming to have the answer to this question but I may have a few clues. Religion

---

is the antidote to doubt, because by definition it requires faith. And doubt is the easiest way to lose one's footing, to slip into unease and anxiety; religion is a safe haven in this uncertain place we call home.

Robertson Davies said, "Fanaticism is ... overcompensation for doubt,"[109] and I agree, as this statement has been proven time and again. When the Hutus in Rwanda slaughtered the Tutsi "cockroaches" they were reacting against seventy years of being told they were lower class, that the Tutsis were their rulers. Historians agree that Hitler's ideology and anti-Semitism grew so quickly in Germany because of the severe economic hardship Germany suffered after WWI. The Germans were forced to sign the Treaty of Versailles and blamed the Jewish community for this, spreading the rumor that high-placed Jewish people, specifically bankers, forced the signing to happen so they could become richer. The rise of the Ku Klux Klan in the early nineteen hundreds was largely a reaction to fears about limited jobs and social change. During a time in history when jobs were scarce, there were large numbers of immigrants from Europe of Jewish and Catholic faith, as well as migrations of African Americans into the Midwest and North. The Klan always grew the most rapidly in cities with high growth rates, finite housing, and fierce competition for jobs. This theme in the rise of fanaticism is constant and speaks more to the human condition than to any ideology or belief system. The bottom line is, when people begin to feel vulnerable they are ripe for manipulation and more easily convinced to perform harmful, even evil acts. This is the opposite of wisdom.

When a person is committed to becoming wiser he works hard to avoid fanaticism in any form, recognizing that it breeds intolerance and ignorance. Examine your most rigidly held ideas and beliefs, especially the ideas that you feel the need to stridently defend. Recognize when you are feeling vulnerable and instead of trying to blame someone for your condition, move into compassion, resilience, and positive change. Few beliefs should be held too tightly; instead they will change over time as you continue to make sense of your life. Wise people recognize that life is full of promise and danger, uncertainty and choice, but they aren't afraid of any of it. They stay clear from dogmatism in any form because they know that it belies personal insight. Life really is, as Walt Whitman says, in his

---

[109] Robertson Davies. (n.d.). Retrieved from http://izquotes.com/quote/47464

poem Song of the Open Road, the long brown path leading wherever I choose.

"Reality is merely an illusion, albeit a very persistent one."
–Albert Einstein[110]

"Row, row, row your boat gently by the stream. Merrily, merrily, merrily, Life is but a dream." These words I sang over and over as a child, not knowing that one day they would become a source of wisdom. Spiritual teachers from a wide range of traditions have long reminded us that we are all living a collective dream. We create our inner world with our mind and thought and we share our outer world through the projected dream we have created. What I've come to realize is that the conscious mind is the storyteller in our life, fabricating the story of our dream. It spends most of its energy trying to explain feelings that we are having and creating stories from them. When we are unaware of the true nature of reality, we take our feelings so much more seriously. They stay with us, are perpetuated, and become embedded in the self-identity we have created. We let the past define the present, and create a present that is prewritten by the storyteller of our mind.

When I was a kid, my Dad would tell me stories about his heroic dog named Wow. I would listen raptly as I heard about Wow the bear chaser, Wow who walked my Dad to school every day and greeted him at the same time every afternoon, Wow who knew every dog trick in the book and could leap tall buildings in a single bound. I imagined having a dog like Wow. In my mind's eye Wow was a huge, bear-like buddy. When I got my first dog Willow, a beautiful golden retriever, I had Wow in mind. One day, on a trip home a few years ago I overheard a conversation between my Dad and my brother. When the name Wow came up, I began to listen intently. My Dad was telling my brother the story of how Wow died. Sadly, my grandmother ran him over with her car as she was backing out of the driveway. "How could she have not seen him?" I asked. "Well he was pretty small. Wow was a Chihuahua. We named him Wow because I called him a chiwowa." I had to laugh. All this time I had created a story of my own about Wow. He had influenced my life, my desire to have a big buddy of my own, but the Wow I had created was a fantasy.

---

[110] Albert Einstein: 10 of his best quotes. (2012, March 30). Retrieved from http://www.telegraph.co.uk/news/science/science-news/9176616/Albert-Einstein-10-of-his-best-quotes.html

Sometimes our storyteller can make us laugh but often it can hold us back, even keeping us sick. In the medical community there are countless accounts of people being diagnosed with an illness, manifesting all the symptoms of the illness, only to find out that they were misdiagnosed. One tragic story from author and MD Michael Crichton, tells of a man who had undergone surgery and was lying in his hospital bed recovering when a group of doctors came in and begin talking. Hearing the words, "dying, just a matter of time, terminal," he was so utterly upset that he ended up passing away the next day. He never found out that they were actually talking about the man in the next bed.

The truth of your life is always evolving. There will be things that you absolutely believe with all your heart until one day you discover that this truth was just something you'd repeated to yourself enough times that you began to believe it. As you move through life the stories build up, evolve, and form the basis for the attitudes and perspectives that shape who you are. It's important to be aware of the stories that have the most influence on you and to occasionally question whether they remain true. If I hadn't questioned whether living with a disease prevented me from being healthy, I never would have written this book. I would never have understood that my health has less to do with the luck of the draw and more to do with the choices I make.

"Not what we have but what we enjoy, constitutes abundance."
–Epicurus[111]

Here is a profound truth: our desires carry with them the heartbeat of our lives. If you honor your desires without struggling to get them they will come to you more easily. Letting go of struggle and worry invokes trust and the knowledge of what true abundance is: having what you need when you need it. Many people forget that we really aren't looking for things; we are looking for feelings. People who desire material things are really desiring love, comfort, security, or connection. Material things can bring us these feelings but only temporarily; like medicine they are band-aides. The real medicine is the source of the feelings they invoke inside us. If

---

[111] Epicurus quote. (n.d.). Retrieved from
http://www.brainyquote.com/quotes/quotes/e/epicurus119455.html

you are clear about what you want, you won't battle with indecision and confuse what abundance really is.

I began to learn this lesson when I was in the fourth grade. This was the first year that fashion was in fashion for the girls in my school and two things were the all the rage: Gloria Vanderbilt jeans and Le Sport Sac purses. For months I watched my lucky classmates come into school prancing in their new jeans or swinging their new purses, and I envied them. If only I had a purse too, my life would be so different. I'd be happier and more grown up; I was convinced life would be much better if only I could join the exclusive jean and purse club. One day my wish came true. I got a blue Le Sport Sac purse for my birthday. When I first opened my present I was giddy with happiness. I spent hours zipping and unzipping each compartment, putting things inside and then taking them out, planning what I would put in my purse for the next day at school.

The next day I walked on cloud nine into the classroom wielding my new purse. One of my schoolmates came up to me and said, "Nice purse!" She then proceeded to show me hers. All of a sudden I felt deflated. I liked hers better: it was cuter, smaller, a neat green instead of boring blue. The immense happiness I felt from my purse lasted less than twenty-four hours before I was back to square one envying yet another item. From that day forward I didn't feel quite as excited about the latest fashion trend. Sure, the day I finally got my Gloria Vanderbilt jeans was a good one, but not a life-changer, and I knew it wouldn't be. Now when I feel a lack in my life, or start to watch as envy creeps in, I ask myself, "Do I have what I need?" Usually the answer is yes, and I can feel content in my abundance. The Stoic philosopher Seneca said, "It is not the man who has little but the man who craves more, that is poor."

There really is no need to struggle ever. Life will at times require a valiant effort, lots of elbow grease and strenuous feats, but struggling will only get in the way of success. Struggling implies a fight, and if you fight life, life will always win. Instead, replace struggle with a conscious effort towards what you truly want. This lends itself to a fortuitous life. For many people this will begin with letting go of worry. Philosopher Alan Watts describes it like this:

> If you feel at this time that an increase in income will solve your problems and you got that increase in income, this would give you a pleasant feeling for a few weeks. But then, as you well know, if that has ever happened to you, the feeling wears off. You may stop worrying about paying your debts and start worrying about whether you will get sick. There is always something to worry about.[112]

Remembering that worry is enemy number one will help a person to replace their anxiety with purposeful dreaming. You never have to earn love, or buy love; you have to shine the light on the love that is already there. This is true for wisdom, health, abundance, and anything else you are striving for. Shining the light on what is already there will allow it to grow.

Self-help gurus love to talk about the power of positive thinking and manifesting what you desire. "Think three positive for every negative thought and you'll be on the way to a new life!" "Create an affirmation and say it out loud as many times as you can throughout the day." "Say, all is well, over and over, and remember you are in charge of your life!" I hear these things and I have to wonder, "How do they know?" I recognize that these platitudes feel really good and are very popular, but to me they ring a bit hollow. Is this lingo wise or just really good marketing? As much as I hate to say it I vote for marketing. The part of me that questions everything in my own search for wisdom realizes that true change requires a lot more than a few well-thought-out phrases repeated 10,000 times. I can tell myself that my body is pain-free and comfortable as much as I want, but this doesn't make it so. After awhile it begins to feel like whistling in the dark.

I'm not saying that positive thinking and affirmations aren't helpful, but they are only tools, not the real alchemy. The alchemy, the miraculous, occurs when you don't turn your back on what you don't like, but instead you embrace the darkness and the light that you hold within. Having conversations with your vulnerable self will teach you much more than ignoring it in favor of staying on a high all the time. When it comes right

---

[112] Watts, A. (1996). Myth and religion: The edited transcripts. (P.4) Boston: Charles E. Tuttle.

down to it we all mostly want the same things: love, comfort, abundance, connection, and to be valued. What makes us interesting is the parts of ourselves that we hide. The parts that struggle with unworthiness, question our ability to ever have the love we crave, or feel like a victim and have begun to lose hope.

So, the next time you think of an affirmation, ask yourself, "Why do I need to say this?" The answer will bring you to the real need. Affirmations are often too directive and come from the ego, not a place of wisdom. Many people turn to affirmations when deep down they feel that something is lacking in their life, when they are seeking to fill a void. Wise people know that understanding how the void was created is vastly more valuable than pretending it's not there.

A compassionate life is a wise one, as long as compassion doesn't morph into idiot compassion. Idiot compassion is a term coined by Tibetan Llama Chögyam Trungpa, and refers to wimpiness disguised as compassion. The motivation behind idiot compassion is the avoidance of conflict and is practiced by people who desire to be seen as nice and good. Idiot compassion perpetuates pain, is spineless, and, well, downright idiotic. Or as Chögyam Trungpa says, "a slimy way of trying to fulfill your desire secretly." He goes on to say:

> Idiot compassion is the highly conceptualized idea that you want to do good. . . . But that doesn't mean to say that you have to be gentle (or presumably nice or kind) all the time. Your gentleness should have heart, strength. In order that your compassion doesn't become idiot compassion (or idiot kindness, or idiot niceness), you have to use your intelligence. Otherwise, there could be self-indulgence of thinking that you are creating a compassionate situation when in fact you are feeding the other person's aggression. If you go to a shop and the shopkeeper cheats you and you go back and let him cheat you again, that doesn't seem to be a very healthy thing to do for others.[113]

You probably wouldn't go back to a shopkeeper who cheats you, but would you go back to a girlfriend who cheats on you? Would you stay with someone who lies to you, saying to yourself, "He

---

[113] Lewis, W. (2012, December 29). Idiot Compassion. Retrieved from http://www.elephantjournal.com/2012/12/idiot-compassion/

screwed up, poor guy just doesn't feel loved; he needs me to show him what love is." Trust is trusting someone to be who they are. It means that you can see clearly that a person who chooses to lie to you lacks personal integrity and if you look the other way because you don't want to rock the boat you are harming yourself and the person who lied. By continuing to trust a person who lies or cheats, you are disrespecting yourself and not giving them the chance to change. What that person really needs is to be called onto the table and held accountable even if what they want is to get away with their bad behavior.

Here is something Buddhist teacher Pema Chodron has to say about this subject:

> ...if someone is violent, for instance, and is being violent towards you ... it's not the compassionate thing to keep allowing that to happen, ... it will be quite difficult for you to go through the process of actually leaving the situation. But that's the compassionate thing to do. It's the compassionate thing to do for yourself, because you're part of that dynamic, and before you always stayed. So now you're going to do something frightening, groundless, and quite different. But it's the compassionate thing to do for yourself, rather than stay in a demeaning, destructive, abusive relationship. And it's the most compassionate thing you can do for them too. They will certainly not thank you for it, and they will certainly not be glad. They'll go through a lot. But if there's any chance for them to wake up or start to work on their side of the problem, their abusive behavior or whatever it might be, that's the only chance, is for you to actually draw the line and get out of there.[114]

A lot of ill health stems from idiot compassion, something I know all too well. For me idiot compassion has been a hard habit to break. It started when I was young, not speaking up and telling the people around me the truth about how I was feeling. Even at a young age I recognized that pain had made me very tough. I could handle much more pain than anyone around me; I was a small girl with a core of steel. I consciously martyred myself, sparing others pain by hurting myself instead, keeping others happy even if I had to suffer in the process. I knew I could handle it but I wasn't sure they could. So

---

[114] Retrieved from: Lewis, W. (2012, December 29). Idiot Compassion. Retrieved from http://www.elephantjournal.com/2012/12/idiot-compassion/

I ended up taking tennis lessons even though they hurt my hands badly because I knew it made my Mom happy. I would go ice-skating on frozen lakes with my friends gritting my teeth the whole time, even though in all likelihood they would have been just as happy if we'd gone swimming instead. Over time, not speaking up about my needs transformed into my not even recognizing what my needs were, let alone if they were being met. This, of course, set me up for decades of unhealthy relationships, all because at the beginning of my life I decided that I didn't want to spoil anyone's day.

What if I hadn't fallen into this trap? Perhaps my ice-skating friends would have learned the art of compromise and my Mom would have been offered the opportunity for a deeper understanding of my pain. Countless boyfriends would have had the opportunity to learn honest communication and empathy. I do know that if I hadn't offered myself on the altar of unnecessary suffering like a sacrificial lamb, I would have had to learn to be tough in a different way. Instead of the little girl who always smiled, winning happiest camper awards at girl- scouts, I would have had to encounter many uncomprehending looks as I explained my situation to the people around me. Maybe there would have been a few accommodations made for me at school and I would have been pegged as different. I would have been physically more isolated but emotionally less so as some of the people around me began to understand. Idiot compassion prevents wisdom from blossoming because it keeps you and the people around you stuck. They never get the opportunity to grow and you, in your perpetual niceness, never develop the strength to stand up for yourself.

Over the years I've learned to trade stoicism for personal integrity. This has allowed me to be less idiot and more compassionate. It hasn't been easy and is something I need to be vigilant with myself about. I continue to be humbled by just how tenaciously this tendency towards idiot compassion has gripped me. But my vigilance has paid off and taught me a few valuable lessons. I've learned that win-win doesn't always mean that both people become happy. Sometimes win-win means that one person stands in their power and another person is given a chance to learn something. I now know that speaking my truth always feels good and swallowing it down eats me up. I've learned that sometimes my job is to plant seeds, and when a loved one is ready for them they will blossom. I've found that integrity is the strength of kings, and stoicism is really just a mask for masochism. Integrity forces you to show up and stoicism allows you to hide. Finally, I've learned that idiot compassion has no use for me anymore.

My Personal Honor Code:

I Will:

- *See others*
- *Listen Well*
- *Trust Myself*
- *Take My Dreams More Seriously and My Life Less Seriously*
- *Have Compassion for Others without taking Responsibility for their Negativity and Suffering*
- *Stop Blaming Myself*
- *Make Decisions that align with my Purpose*
- *Believe in my ability to Heal myself and those around me*
- *Be Spirited, Generous, and Caring*

Creating a personal honor code has been one of the most important things I've ever done. It has helped me to understand myself, what I came here to do, and who I came here to be. It has also greatly improved my personal integrity which is achieved when thoughts, words, and deeds reflect values. I know that if I simply live the principles that reflect my truth I will touch the lives of those I am destined to touch and the doors I am supposed to open will unlock for me. One truth for me is the knowledge that although I don't have the authority to stand in judgment of others, I have the responsibility to hold myself accountable for my actions. An unexamined life is a wasted one. My personal honor code has created a framework from which I live. It allows me to see when I veer off track and as I reign myself back in gives me insights when I ask myself the question, "Why exactly did I do that?" It has helped me to know myself. My honor code is the source of my authenticity and it shows me how to make choices that empower me. It sometimes morphs and changes as I grow, but the core of it remains unchanged. It has taken me out of my comfort zone as I have realized that the life I chose had more to do with what was expected of me than what I freely chose for myself. It has made me more honest with myself and others.

"The reason why many are still troubled, still seeking, still making little forward progress is because they haven't yet come to the end of themselves. We're still trying to give orders, and interfering with God's work within us." –A.W. Tozer[115]

Before I was ready to create and live my personal honor code I had to stop telling life what I wanted from it. Instead, I learned to listen and let my life speak to me. Then I had to accept what I heard. We offer so much energy resisting what is, wanting to be something or someone different. We can resist all we want, but we won't be able to change the truth of what is. Surrendering to what is can be one of the most powerful things you'll ever do on behalf of yourself. The trick is to avoid surrendering to a situation that is culturally defined. Instead, surrender as a free and independent human being, accepting the person behind the mask that society has created. In my case I had to accept that, like it or not, I have lived with a disease that has been named rheumatoid arthritis for most of my life. Obviously not something I would have chosen, but the more I try to subdue it, deny it, or judge it, the more it consumes me. I recognize that rheumatoid arthritis is just a label, created by the modern medical community to describe a cluster of symptoms. I also understand that my experience of this cluster of symptoms is both similar to and entirely unique from others with the same label. I have my own experiences, DNA, and emotional life. So my life speaks to me in a singular way, just as it does for everyone else.

As I described earlier in the book, when I humbled myself enough to let my life speak I realized that my mind had crippled me much more than my body. I'd let the word cripple haunt me and skew how I viewed myself as I looked at my less-than-perfect body. I compared myself to others who I viewed as more physically perfect, not realizing that those people were comparing themselves to other, more "perfect" people still. I didn't understand that focusing on physical or material perfection is an endless black hole that never satisfies because there will always be someone better looking, healthier, or wealthier than you. I was living blind to the reality that trying to be the perfect one only served to distance me from the truth that we are all one. What really cripples a person isn't their

---

[115] Warren, Rick. "Come To The End Of Yourself." *Come To The End Of Yourself*. N.p., 21 May 2014. Web. 29 May 2015.

body, or their circumstance; it is their mind and judgment. When I finally understood this I was free to let my life speak. As you learn to do this, you will find that your wisdom grows.

"Child's mind is Buddha's mind. Just seeing, just doing is truth. Then, using this mind means when you are hungry, eat. When someone is hungry, give them food." - Soen Sa Nim[116]

Wise people maintain what is called in Buddhism, the child's, or beginner's, mind. They know that if a belief system no longer works for them it is best to throw it out and change. They also know that, like a snake shedding its skin, getting rid of old belief systems is a requirement for personal growth. I no longer believe the Nike saying, "No pain no gain," or that pushing myself through severe pain is always the best option. If I did, I wouldn't be as healthy as I am.

The other thing that maintaining a child's mind does for you is help you to avoid over-thinking things. Remember, the age group with the highest survival rate when lost in nature is people under six. Six-year-olds won't try to out-smart Mother Nature and will always take care of their immediate needs first. They won't tell themselves, "If I take a nap right now I'm being lazy; I should just keep going until I'm done." How many times have you told yourself this and ended up completely screwing up your task? I've broken glasses trying to clean the kitchen when I was tired, put things away and immediately forgot where I put them, and forgotten all my important items at the grocery store, all because I refused to listen to my body's need for rest. If you can master the art of staying present and doing what needs to be done without prejudgment, you are moving into the wisdom of the child's mind.

I once heard a story from my tai chi instructor that is a Zen proverb called "A cup of tea." It goes like this:

One day a Japanese master had a visit from a university professor. The professor wanted to learn about the way of Zen. The master poured the professor a cup of tea. As he was pouring, he didn't stop, letting the cup overflow. The professor watched and finally burst out, " It is too full, you are letting the tea spill out!" The Japanese master replied," You are like this

---

[116] Sahn, S. (n.d.). Child's Mind is Buddha's Mind | Kwan Um School of Zen. Retrieved from http://www.kwanumzen.org/?teaching=childs-mind-is-buddhas-mind

cup- so full of your own opinions and ideas. I cannot show you Zen until you empty your cup."

Most adults I know are guilty of full-cup syndrome. We've already got it figured out and our ideas shape our views. We think we are being intelligent and logical, but in fact we are being close-minded and irrational. Tell an ardent Democrat or Republican that their decision to back their candidate is an emotional, not rational one, and they will most likely, with high emotion, disagree.

Ninety percent of decisions are based on emotion. This isn't necessarily a bad thing. The emotional system has evolved over millennia and is a fine-tuned instrument, but it is also highly influenced by past experiences, especially negative ones. Understanding this will help you to consciously work with your emotions. Did you grow up with a mother who watched what you ate like a hawk, criticizing you for eating sweets? Is this why eating a cookie makes you anxious and causes you to surreptitiously eat ten when all you wanted was one? How many relationships have been tainted by old "baggage"? Living wisely involves consciously engaging in each new situation with the child's mind, free of pre-judgment. Take the lessons of the past with you but don't let them strangle the present.

"Chance only favours the mind which is prepared."
– Louis Pasteur[117]

The mundane aspects of life, the everyday interactions with others, remain mundane until you bring awareness to the table. The ability to be purposeful in your interactions makes every single thing you do meaningful. You create what you want by focusing on solutions, not problems, by remaining open to endless possibilities, by remembering that you usually have to come to a few closed doors until you find the open one, by learning to shift your perspective, and by letting go of how you receive your solutions. I was reminded of this not too long ago during an all-too-familiar experience for many of us. I was flying across the country and found myself in the longest customer service line I had ever seen after my flight got canceled. As one could imagine, my first reaction was utter

---

[117] Barnett, B. (n.d.). Louis Pasteur: Chance Favors the Prepared Mind. Retrieved from http://www.pasteurbrewing.com/articles/life-of-pasteur/louis-pasteur-chance-favors-prepared-mind/173.html

irritation and dismay. I looked at the line again, stopped myself, and realized that if I kept feeling this way I'd be irritated for an extremely long time. So I started a conversation with the woman in front of me. We quickly got beyond the, "Where are you from, where are you going," stage of idle chitchat and began to talk about our lives. Before long I had learned a lot, gained some inspiration, and made a new friend. Once you attain the habit of remembering how you want to be, circumstance doesn't have to change this. And you will find much wisdom along the way.

I once heard a Taoist story from my Tai Chi instructor that I won't soon forget. There was an old farmer who had a horse to work his crops. One day the horse went missing. Upon hearing this his neighbors stopped by and said, "My, what a horrible situation." The farmer replied, "Maybe." The next day the horse returned with three other wild horses. His neighbors once again visited. "Wow, how amazing, you are so lucky!" they exclaimed. "Maybe," said the farmer. The following day his only son attempted to ride one of the wild horses, was bucked off, and broke his leg. "I'm so sorry for you," said his neighbors, "Without your son to help you will have much difficulty keeping the farm going." "Maybe," was once again the reply. Soon thereafter military officials came to their small town drafting all the young men for the army.

The persistent, yet apparently dimwitted neighbors, once again stopped by. "Congratulations!" they said. "Maybe," the farmer replied. If there ever was a better demonstration that you should never get too caught up in the so-called victories and defeats of life, I haven't heard it. Whatever your current situation, try saying, "This too shall pass." Or perhaps, "Savor the moment," depending on what is going on!

Sometimes the irony of life can make you shake your head. The fact is that life is change. Challenges will lead to good times, and even if they don't they will bring personal growth and wisdom. The "good" and "bad" things we experience are equally valuable and must be similarly honored and even cherished no matter how bad they seem at the time. When life doesn't happen the way you envisioned or planned it's best to open your mind and ask yourself, "I wonder what's coming next?" Often the answer will be way beyond the limited capacity of your imagination, regardless of how creative it is. You will transform your plight into an exciting journey, and the book of your life will become a page-turner instead of a boring textbook.

"Knowledge is learning something every day. Wisdom is letting go of something every day." – Zen Proverb[118]

Wisdom and healing have something in common: they both are more about letting go than adding. This isn't widely understood; modern medicine certainly hasn't figured this one out. Instead, people searching to heal themselves are counseled to add medicine, surgeries, treatments, new diets, supplements; once you are diagnosed with an illness you will immediately be presented with a mind-boggling to-do list. No wonder so many people go into denial and sink further into themselves. Letting go of what no longer serves you will move a person into health so much quicker than trying to add something that never belonged to you in the first place. Instead, it belongs to someone, however well meaning, who never walked in your shoes. The same is true for wisdom. Learning the ideas of others may make you smart, but it will never make you wise. Whenever you are in need of healing or wisdom, ask, "What can I let go?" It might be an unhelpful emotion, a responsibility that you don't really need to take on, a self-expectation, or all of the above. By first letting go you will free your body, mind, and spirit to bring forth the true wisdom and healing it needs.

"A kind soul is in constant bloom." - A.D. Williams[119]

When I think about truly wise people, one characteristic that they share is an innate kindness. I think this kindness emanates so strongly from them because they have mastered compassion, a humble attitude, and the knowledge that kindness is really the only healthy way to approach life. Kindness is rarely met with resistance, and it always brings good feeling. Innate kindness can only be attained when a person lets go of fear. The character who most epitomizes this for me is Ebenezer Scrooge. Most of us know the story of the tight-fisted, cold-hearted man who dismissed the spirit of Christmas with a disgustful "Bah-humbug!" Mr. Scrooge is the richest man in town but won't lend a penny to a needy soul, and even goes so far as saying that the poor may be better off dying so as to "decrease the surplus population." He treats his only

[118] A Quote by Zen Proverb on wisdom, knowledge, learning, letting go, and zen. (n.d.). Retrieved from http://blog.gaiam.com/quotes/authors/zen-proverb/61851
[119] Retrieved From: http://jeannesblissblog.blogspot.com/2014/02/we-are-here-to-heal-not-harm.html

employee, Bob Cratchit, like dirt, and his one concession to a semblance of kindness is to give Mr. Cratchit Christmas day off. As the story of this most hateful character progresses, however, he emerges as a very sad man.

He hoards his money and lives in a hovel. He denies not only those around him but also himself. He does this because he was never able to move beyond the fears that engulfed him in childhood. When Scrooge was a baby his mother died and he had to live on the streets. Books were his only companions. Scrooge was finally invited back to live with his father but soon thereafter his father went to jail for not paying a debt. Scrooge became obsessed with making money, to the detriment of the rest of his life. He lost his fiancé due to his greed, which put the final stone in place for him and sealed his fate.

Scrooge's fear of losing the only thing he had, money, ruled his life and made him a miserable, mean miser until the fateful night when he was visited by the three spirits of Christmas: Past, Present, and Future. The night ended with Scrooge shedding his fear and opening his heart to his biggest fear: other people. Once his fear was conquered, kindness emerged. Here is how the Dickens book ends:

> Some people laughed to see the alteration in him, but he let them laugh, and little heeded them; for he was wise enough to know that nothing ever happened on this globe, for good, at which some people did not have their fill of laughter at the outset; and knowing that such as these would be blind anyway, he thought it quite as well that they should wrinkle up their eyes in grins, as have the malady in less attractive forms. His own heart laughed and that was quite enough for him.[120]

If there was ever a better story of true transformation into kindness I haven't heard it.

Author and spiritual teacher Caroline Myss says that fear brings fate, and freedom from fear brings destiny. When Scrooge let his fear go he unsealed his fate as a lonely, mean, sad old man and instead became a man with endless opportunities for connection and true happiness. Anyone who has seen the movie A Christmas Carol sees a man at the end of the movie who is finally comfortable in his own skin. He has the

---

[120] Retrieved from: http://en.wikiquote.org/wiki/A_Christmas_Carol

ability to be kind because he is no longer torturing himself with his unmet yearnings. Although it is hard to admit, most of us have a bit of Scrooge hanging out inside. We choose to seal fates of different kinds out of fear in many ways. It can be a job that you stay with because it has good benefits even though going to work every day makes you feel twenty times heavier. Or being afraid to move on from an unhealthy relationship because you are afraid of being alone. Or being afraid to commit to a relationship. It could be never spending that three months in the Caribbean learning to sail even though you had the time and money because you were afraid others might call you irresponsible. There are endless ways each of us find to seal our fates, which in the end limits us in ways we may never know. Oliver Wendell Holmes said, "Most people go to their grave with their music inside them."[121]

The search for wisdom always brings you back to yourself. It begins with the decision to never stop learning, grows with dogged determination, and is embedded over time into the person you become. Wisdom breeds curiosity which in turn leads to further wisdom; there is no destination, only more learning. "The growth of the human mind," Norman Cousins says, "is a high adventure, in many ways the highest adventure on earth."[122] If we always remember that this life is an endless opportunity we will continue to experiment, and not waste any occasion we have to become a healthier, more content human being.

[121] "Oliver Wendell Holmes, Sr. Quote." *BrainyQuote*. Xplore, n.d. Web. 29 May 2015.
[122] "Norman Cousins." *Iz Quotes*. n.d. Web. 29 May 2015.

EPILOGUE
"Hurt or Heal?"

Who am I really? Am I my disease, am I the things that I do, the religion that I follow? Am I where I work, the family I grew up in, the state that I spent my early years? Am I my country? Am I my body, my emotions, my thoughts? Am I healthy or am I ill? Am I who I want to be? Am I who I'm capable of being? Am I taking responsibility for the person I've become? Am I living an authentic life? Am I filled with fear or love, judgment or compassion, knowledge or wisdom? When I wake up in the morning do I shine the light on health or illness? Do I walk through life with wonder or frustration?

Every minute of every day the decisions you make and the actions you take guide whether you will continue to hurt or move into healing. Other people can help you to tip the scale in one direction or the other, but ultimately health is an inside job. You fight pain by showing up as yourself, 110%, every day, regardless of what your external circumstances are reflecting, despite what your past conditioning has told you about who you are.

The path to health is unique for everyone, but will incorporate belief in oneself and the ability to heal, a purpose as a sense of energy and direction, the ability to be a maverick, honesty with oneself and others, putting forth true effort every day, honoring the movement of the body and the rhythms of life, unlearning unresilience, honoring and meeting the body's needs, giving the gift of love every day, fostering genuine connection, learning to walk with pain, strengthening spirit, and continuously seeking wisdom.

Committing to true health with a full heart and unfettered integrity will change you forever. Although there are no guarantees in life, this I can say: Life really is beautiful, all you need to do is open your eyes and see.

BOOK
DISCUSSION
QUESTIONS

BELIEF

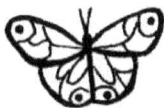

1. The author has some very strong words about the modern medical system, stating that it is as ill as the people it treats- do you agree with this? Why or Why not?
2. How has the modern medical approach to illness affected the way you think about your health or disease?
3. What have you chosen to believe about your disease?
4. Do you believe in yourself and your ability to heal?
5. Take some time to ponder the following questions, and answer them as honestly as possible:
    a. Is my body capable of more than I give it credit for?
    b. What have I been told about myself that isn't true?
    c. What have I been told about my disease?
    d. What is my disease telling me?
    e. Am I living the life that I think I should have or the one I want?
    f. How do my beliefs make me feel?
    g. Have I given up on any beliefs because of the influence of others?
    h. Who and what has influenced my beliefs about myself?
6. The author says that our beliefs create the fabric of our life; if this is true, by looking at your life, can you think of which beliefs have influenced you the most?
7. The author talks about her struggle with hope; is this something you can relate to? If so, how can you take the first step, as she did, to keep hope alive and move towards health?

PURPOSE

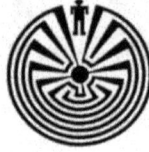

1. What is your life purpose?

   In reflecting on your own special purpose it is helpful to ask yourself some questions:

   a. Who were you at the age of twelve? What did you enjoy doing, what were your hobbies, your interests, and your dreams? At this age most people haven't yet been too corrupted by their inner judge or by societies' expectations.
   b. Who most inspires you? Who do you look at and see qualities that motivate and impress you?
   c. What do your friends and family ask you for assistance with?
   d. What things make you the happiest?
   e. What can you do everyday and never get tired of?
   f. What are you doing when you lose track of time?
   g. What do you deeply believe in?
   h. What ideas are you the most passionate about?
   i. If you could clone yourself what would your clone be doing right now?
   j. What have been the most challenging episodes in your life? How did you move past them? What did you learn from them?
   k. Where does the majority of your suffering come from? Can you find meaning in this suffering? How can you use this to help others?
   l. What has your life experience taught you? How can this unique experience help others?
   m. What are your greatest talents and skills?
   n. What are your most cherished values?
   o. How do you most want to be of service for the greater good?

2. What has your disease taught you about your purpose?

3. Reflect on Frankl's three tenets of Logotherapy: Freedom of will, Will to meaning, and Meaning of life. How can you apply them to your life right now?

4. Write a personal mission statement and refer to it regularly, especially when you are making life decisions.

MAVERICK

決心

1. Have you ever been bullied into making a medical decision that you didn't feel good about? What was the outcome? How will you prevent this from happening again?

2. Can you think of a time when your medical treatment has been compassionate? How did that make you feel?

3. What does your inner guidance tell you is best for your health right now? Is there one thing you can do that will honor that guidance?

4. What were your childhood dreams? Which ones came to fruition? Are there any dreams that you can fulfill now?

5. Who is your favorite maverick?

6. What aspects of yourself are you not willing to give up because of your illness?

7. What parts of your illness do you keep to yourself?

8. Where do you find your joy? What makes you happy to be alive?

9. Are you reactive or proactive in your response to your disease? Where are you reactive and where are you pro-active? How can you encourage yourself to be more pro-active?

HONESTY

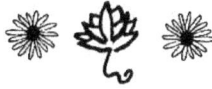

1. Do you see evidence of the post-truth society that the author talks about in your own life experience? Where is it most prominent?

2. What are you hungry for? Where are you vulnerable to being lied to? Are you hungry for money, fame, prestige, respect, admiration, love, feeling desired?

3. Reflect on the three enemies to honesty that the author mentions: Justification, Ego, and Rigid Thinking. Are any of these traits that you need to work on? How can you begin to be more honest with yourself around the ways that you deflect self-truth?

4. Have you ever lived through a situation where you found yourself or someone you know justify their bad behavior? What was the result? How would the situation have turned out differently if the truth was told?

5. Are there any hurtful truths you've avoided telling yourself or others? Can you think of a loving way to tell the truth next time it comes up?

6. Can you commit to right speech? Try it on for 1 week and see what happens.

7. Who is the most honest person you know? How is their life different from the less honest people you know? What one thing can you do today to emulate their commitment to honesty?

EFFORT

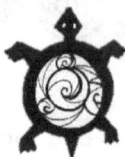

1. Does your life right now reflect more of the hamster-on-the-wheel effort or true effort?

2. Where do you waste effort?

3. In what areas of your life can you put forth more effort?

4. In what areas of your life is remaining unattached to the outcome the most difficult? How can you change this?

5. Reflect on the Dalai Lama quote mentioned in this chapter, "If you think you can't make a difference try sleeping with a mosquito." Can you think of a time when a small action or decision on your part had a much larger impact than you anticipated? Does this encourage you to do more small gestures throughout your day?

6. Create a vision board and let your intention guide your efforts

MOVEMENT

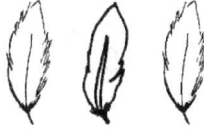

1. Do you make moving your body part of your everyday life? If not why not? How can you encourage yourself to start doing this?

2. How do you handle the ups and downs of your disease or life challenges? Do you help yourself to create ease when life challenges you or do you fight what is happening?

3. The author talks about the phrase, "You can only lean one way at once." Can you go through one day and observe which way you are leaning, and then begin to choose a more helpful response the next time you find yourself leaning into a harmful reaction?

4. What small shift can you create today that will help you move into a more healthy lifestyle?

5. Do you hold onto your emotions and feelings after they no longer serve you? If so, how can you begin to let them move through you more quickly?

6. Do your thoughts create resistance to what is happening in your life? How can you shift this pattern?

RESILIENCE

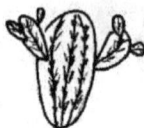

1. Take some time to go out in nature and notice examples of resilience- what do they teach you about your own life and situation?

2. Which of your family and friends encourage feelings of resilience in you, and help you to be resilient? Do you encourage resilience in others?

3. Do you feel that you persevere during challenging times or are you quick to give up? How can you do better next time?

4. In the past have you judged your failures as an end or, can you say, as Thomas Edison did, "I haven't failed, I've identified 10,000 ways this doesn't work."

5. How can you acknowledge and celebrate the small steps you are taking to live well?

6. Take time to think about a challenge you are experiencing right now and create a mantra to help you shift your perspective around it.

7. What are your biggest fears and why? Are your fears keeping you from being resilient? Are they helping you or keeping you stuck?

8. Are you in survival mode right now? If so, how can you get out of it? Pick a stress relieving activity and incorporate it onto your daily routine.

SELF-CARE

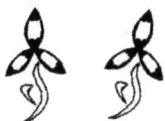

1. How you can begin to take steps to be your own best friend?

2. What are the motives that have driven your behavior and shaped your life? How many of them are motives that come from your own desires, not from your upbringing or society?

3. Are there any unhealthy beliefs about yourself you carry which are shaping your behavior right now?

4. How many hours of sleep does your body need to feel good? Are you honoring that need?

5. Do you move your body every day? If not why not? Can you make an action plan today to move more often?

6. Do you eat with a good attitude? If not, where do your unhelpful thoughts around eating come from and how can you change them?

7. How can you increase the pleasure in your life? What pleasurable activities can you begin to incorporate into your life on a regular basis?

LOVE

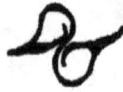

1. How can you love yourself more?

2. Which of the three quotes by Osho, Jesus, or Don Miguel Ruiz resonates most with you? Find a quote about love that you like and place it somewhere that you see often.

3. Do you believe in your inherent worth? If the answer is no, can you find aspects of yourself that can increase your feelings of worthiness?

4. Are your closest relationships mirroring your own patterns of self-abuse? If so, are you willing to change this?

5. What traits do you have that you are proud of? What do you shine at? Are you showing these traits to the world or are you hiding them?

6. Are you able to forgive yourself and the people that have hurt you? If not, what can you do to take a step towards forgiveness? Can your compassion begin to over-ride your need to assign fault?

7. Do you know anyone who has sunk into apathy? What can you do to help them move back towards love?

CONNECTION

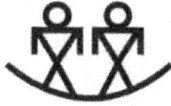

1. How connected do you feel to your family, friends, and community? Is there a way you can foster more support?

2. Refer to the Worksheet on the next page entitled, "Your Go-To-Crew" and fill it out. Use the people on your list to foster the support you need.

3. If you or someone you love has a chronic disease, does the other person feel like a caregiver? How can you shift that relationship into a more balanced one? Can you try to model the relationship a bit more like the one Bonnie and Mark have in the book?

4. Is there anyone who you have true companionship with, who is able to sit with you without judgment during the darkest times in your life? If so, write them a thank-you letter. If not, become that person for someone else and you will find it.

5. How good are you at asking for support when you need it? If you know you will pay it forward later does that lift your reluctance?

MY GO-TO-CREW

Who can bring me comfort when I'm down, and provide the emotional support that I need?

_____

_____

_____

_____

Who makes me laugh? Who can I call when I just need to lighten up?

_____

_____

_____

Who helps me to relax?

_____

_____

_____

Who motivates me?

_____

_____

_____

Who can help me to problem-solve?

_____

_____

_____

PAIN

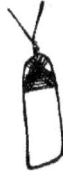

1. Do you deal with daily physical or emotional pain? What is your current way that you deal with it? Do you have any strategies that decrease your pain? If so, do you practice them regularly?

2. What thoughts come up when your pain gets bad? Do they make your pain better or worse?

3. Have you ever been disappointed because of magical thinking? In your life now do you fall prey to magical thinking? If so how can you turn those thoughts into more realistic, yet hopeful ones?

4. How do you compound your pain by fighting against it? Can you just let it be without judgment and see what happens?

5. Has your inner guidance ever helped you deal with a painful situation? What was the result?

6. Do you or anyone you know have aspects of the walking wounded?

7. Do you recognize that, as Maria Shriver said, "Life is a marathon, not a race?" If not, how can you be more patient with yourself?

8. When you are in pain can you accept your present circumstance and then willfully but patiently, take steps to help yourself? Can you do this for others?

9. Has your pain changed your personality? How can you start to take steps to let the real you begin to emerge again?

SPIRIT

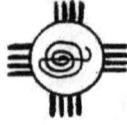

1. What do you think of when you hear the word Spirituality?

2. How do you experience spirituality in your daily life?

3. Consider the four aspects of experiencing spirituality that Deepak Chopra talks about: Being, Feeling, Thinking, and Doing. Which if any of them are you consciously working with right now to enhance your spiritual life? Are there any others that would be helpful to you right now?

4. Do you remember a time when your spirit was able to infuse you with hope or the energy to persevere in times of severe challenge?

5. How does your spirit communicate with you: prayer, meditation, dreams, gut feelings? Something else, or all of the above? Is there a way you can enhance this communication?

6. Do you believe that you are given only what you can handle? If not what do you believe?

7. What difficult lessons have you learned during your life that have later inspired you or enabled you to inspire others?

8. Do you respect your inner wisdom? Why or why not?

9. How comfortable are you with change?

10. What happens when you quiet your mind? What activities enhance this ability for you? How often do you do them?

WISDOM

1. Can you think of one piece of wisdom that your life has taught you that you have been able to help others with?

2. Who is the wisest person you know? What traits do they possess?

3. Have you ever fallen prey to dogmatic thinking? How has this thinking affected your health?

4. Have you ever experienced something like the Wow story in the book, where you misheard or misunderstood something and it affected how you behaved? How did learning the accurate story affect you?

5. Can you think of a story that you have told yourself, which continues to perpetuate a negative dynamic in your life? Ask yourself if it's really true and if the answer is no, begin to change the story to a more helpful one. Watch as your life and relationships change.

6. Do you believe, as the author does, that abundance is having what you need when you need it? If so do your actions and life reflect this believe?

7. Are there any parts of yourself that you find hard to accept? What would happen if you began to accept them now, and began the search for understanding how they emerged in the first place? The author mentions unworthiness, unlovable, being a victim, and hopelessness as negative beliefs that people struggle with; what can you add to this list for yourself?

8. In your own life, how often are you on the receiving end of true compassion versus sympathy? How often are you truly compassionate?

9. Is idiot compassion something you relate to? If so how can you change this tendency? Can you pick one situation that you are in right now or have been in

recently that you were practicing idiot compassion? What could you have differently in this situation?

10. What is your personal honor code?

11. Right now, how many of your actions reflect your values?

12. Do you have more of a child's mind, as described in the book, or full cup syndrome?

13. In the book the author describes standing in line at the airport, how she changed her perspective and made it a positive experience. Is there a situation that you've experienced lately that would have benefited from you doing this as well? Or were you able to change your perspective and improve a situation for yourself?

14. Who is the kindest person you know? Do they have traits of wisdom as well?

15. Reflect on the traits of wise people listed in the beginning of the chapter. Which ones can you begin to enhance in yourself? What traits can you add to the list?